THE ENCYCLOPEDIA OF
ENERGY
HEALING

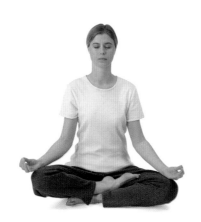

THE ENCYCLOPEDIA OF
ENERGY HEALING

A COMPLETE GUIDE TO USING THE MAJOR FORMS OF HEALING FOR THE BODY, MIND, AND SPIRIT

ANDY BAGGOTT

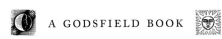 A GODSFIELD BOOK

Library of Congress Cataloging-in-Publication Data Available

10 9 8 7 6 5 4 3 2 1

Published in 1999 by Sterling Publishing Company, Inc.
387 Park Avenue South, New York, N.Y. 10016
© 1999 Godsfield Press
Text © 1999 Andy Baggott
Andy Baggott asserts the moral right to be identified as the author of this work.

Distributed in Canada by Sterling Publishing
c/o Canadian Manda Group, One Atlantic Avenue, Suite 105 Toronto, Ontario, Canada M6K 3E7
Distributed in Australia by Capricorn Link (Australia) Pty Ltd
PO Box 6651, Baulkham Hills, Business Centre, NSW 2153, Australia

Printed and bound in Hong Kong

Sterling ISBN 0-8069-9907-1

With thanks to
Emma Allard, Sapphire Allard, Lucie Allen, Genevieve Applebee, Ian Appleyard, Neil Bell, Alex Bill, Emma Barthes, Sonia Blakely, Duncan Blinkhorn, Linda Bridgeford, Tina Bridgman, Hanna Burchell, Gary Carter, James Cheung, R. J. Clarke, Annie Ferguson, Simon Garrett, Sylvia Gibbons, Denise Hammond, L. Hill, Rosemary Hobbs, Peter Hoggarth, P. Hoksbergen, Katie Howell, Saskia Jackson, Patricia James, Alfred Johnson, Lucianne Lassalle, Marianna Lassalle, Alison Lee-Eyre, Jane Manze, Mike Merchant, Frankie Morrice, Atsuo Murakami, C. Oxley, Manjit Pabla, Ian Preston, Viola Santing, R. Wilding, Marek Urbanowiez, Philippa Vaughan
for help with photography

With thanks to:
Cargo Homeshop, Brighton and The Plinth Company, Stowmarket, Suffolk
for the kind loan of props

PICTURE CREDITS

Abode: p. 183c.
AKG London: p. 67t.
Art Directors & TRIP Photo Library: pp.13t, 44, 51r, 63tr, 78tr, 87, 114, 122bc, 166l, 167tr, 167b, 179 (both), 182br, 186bc, 188b.
A–Z Botanical: pp. 147c, 166b, 168t, 168cr 168b.
Bridgeman Art Library: pp. 15t, 42b, 122bl, 165tl, 170t, 186br.
British Aikido Federation: pp. 94t, 95t.
Bruce Coleman: pp. 140 (both), 148tl.
Christie's Image: p. 171t.
CORBIS: pp. 95, /Austrian Archives p. 188t; /Bettmann pp. 154–5; /Jerry Cooke: p. 21; /Owen Franken: p.91t; /Kimbell Art Museum: p. 165br; /Stephanie Maze: p. 152bl; /Kevin R. Morris: p. 88tr; /Paul A. Souders: p. 86.
e.t. archive: pp. 42t, 116b, 146, 149. 165bl.
Eye Ubiquitous: p. 141.
Garden Picture Library: pp. 167tl, 183t.

George Ohsawa Macrobiotic Foundation: p. 70tl.
Images Colour Library: pp. 11, 12, 15b, 16bl, 26, 35bl, 35br, 43bl, 45tr, 50, 56r, 59bc, 59br, 65t, 71, 78tl, 82b, 96b, 133t, 163tr, 165tr, 180b, 186tr, 189.
London Flotation Centre: pp. 80–1.
Mary Evans Picture Library: p. 108t.
Peter Newark's Pictures: p. 152t.
Dr Randolph Stone: p. 113tl.
Rex Features: p. 62.
Science Photo Library: pp. 13b, 14, 20, 32, 36, 41, 47l, 48, 49b, 59bl, 76b, 79t, 82t, 115t, 116cl, c and cr, 117bl, 124, 126, 130t, 133c, 138tl, 139t, 139b, 142b, 145t, 147t, 152br, 164, 168cl, 169t, 176tr, 177t (deadly nightshade), 178, 182bl, 183t.
Tony Stone Images: pp. 55, 72b, 79b, 115b, 120t, 128t, 131t, 133b, 137, 170b, 173b, 185.
The Wellcome Centre Medical Photographic Library: p. 118t.
Werner Forman Archive: p. 171b.

Contents

Introduction

The Western interest in alternative and complementary therapies is growing almost daily. Many people are searching for answers to their health problems, be they physical, emotional, or spiritual, which Western medicine and religion seem unable to provide. This search inevitably leads them into the realm of energy and energy healing. Because the realm of energy healing is inhabited by human beings, it is like any other area of life, a mixture of good and not so good – there are some low quality therapists in virtually every field of alternative medicine.

This book is designed to allow searchers to find good therapists and to inspire therapists to be high quality practitioners. It looks at the basic concepts behind energy and energy healing, showing which universal qualities make for high quality energy healing. You will be encouraged to experience this "energy" firsthand and to learn how to perceive the energy of other people and potential practitioners. With expert advice on what makes a good therapist in all the major fields of alternative medicine, you will be able to explore this vast and fascinating realm in safety. The first part of the book also discusses and compares Western and Eastern concepts of energy and health, showing how much of our modern lifestyle is contributing to our ill health.

The second part provides a comprehensive encyclopedia of energy healing, explaining what each therapy is and telling you how to find a high quality practitioner. Wherever possible, exercises and information are included to allow you to experience therapies firsthand before deciding whether they are right for you or not. Energy is something you have to experience for yourself to fully understand it.

How to use this book

This book can be used in a variety of ways. If read cover to cover, it will provide you with a firm grounding in all the major concepts of energy and energy healing. It discusses concepts that may well be new to many readers, whether they are novices or experienced practitioners, because the emphasis throughout is on what makes high quality healing and how you can experience high quality living.

This book can also be used as a reference work because it provides grounding in all the major alternative therapies and the concepts of energy that they are built on. It can also be "dipped" into because it is designed to be a book of truths. This means that every page is filled with tangible facts about energy and energy healing, which can be used to improve your quality of life. It is highly illustrated, allowing you to use all of your senses to build up a picture in your mind of this fascinating and potentially life-changing subject.

However you use this book, remember that its intention is to bring about harmony and love. I trust that you will find it enlightening and inspiring.

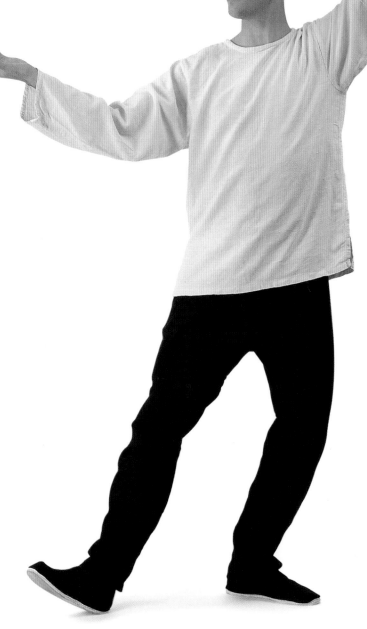

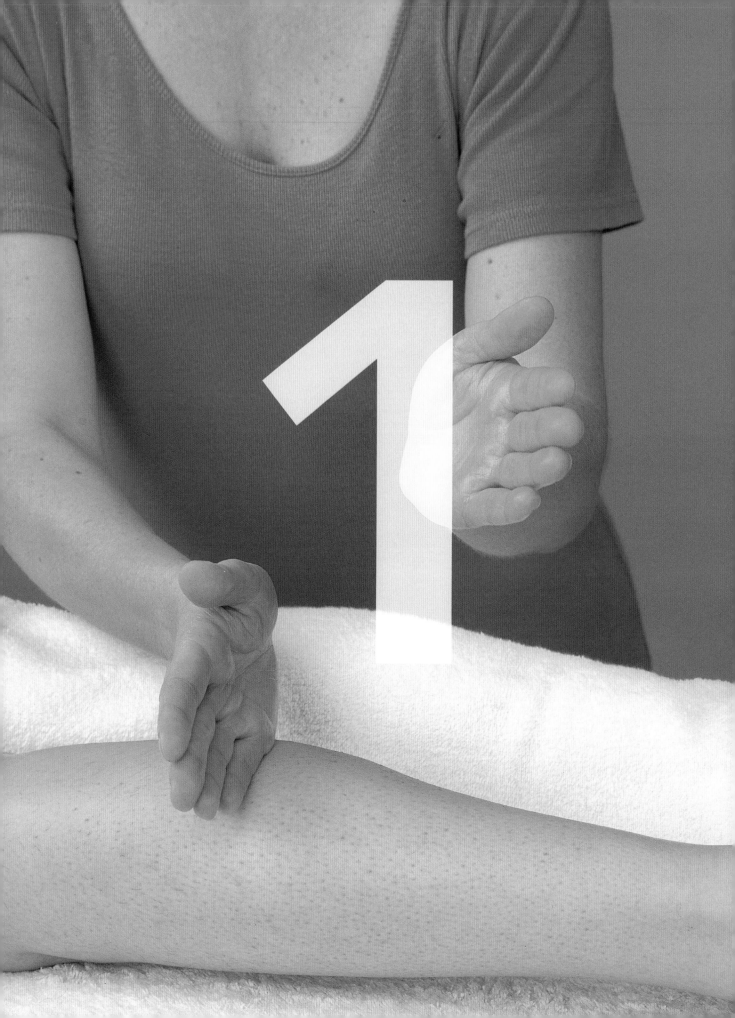

energy healing

There are fundamental truths on which our "understanding" of the universe is founded. These truths are not dependent on science, religion, or any other thought pattern; they just are! One of these truths is that everything in the universe is an expression of energy or, put another way, nothing that exists is devoid of energy. Even the atoms that make up this printed page have energy in a state of dynamic equilibrium. As human beings we have a great deal of this "energy," which often causes us to lose our sense of equilibrium. This leads to "dis-ease" or disharmony and it is then that we need energy healing – any form of action that helps to restore "ease" and harmony to an individual.

Who needs energy healing? Everyone could benefit from some form of energy healing. We thrive on interaction with other humans throughout our lives. The parent who cuddles their upset child is giving energy healing. People who put themselves out for the sake of another are giving energy healing. In one sense, each and every one of us is an energy healer.

Sometimes, when we lose our sense of harmony, nothing we do seems to restore it. This is the time to seek energy healing. The type of energy healing you look for will depend on the cause of your disharmony. You could seek a practitioner or learn to heal yourself by attending a class. The important thing is to seek. Christ, when he said, "Seek and you will find" was speaking a universal truth.

The more you understand a subject, the better you will be able to assess its worth, and this is true of energy and energy healing. In the following chapters, we will discover what energy is and how it works in our daily lives, and you will see how energy healing works. If a particular method of healing appeals to you, it has significance in your life, and will be part of the answer you are seeking to the questions that life is posing you.

1 understanding energy

The universe is made up of many different types of energy. Heat and light are two of the fundamental energies needed to support life. The food we eat has an energy that we convert into life force to feed our bodies. Every thought and action is a form of energy and all of the different forms of energy we come into contact with in our daily lives have an influence on us.

Perceiving energy

Just because you cannot see a particular type of energy does not mean that it doesn't exist. Fire is a form of energy, so are the waves in the sea – both are very easy to perceive. But what about microwaves, radio waves, and radiation? You cannot see the energy entering your television set or radio, but that does not mean that you refuse to use it. You cannot see radiation emanating from the sun but that does not mean that you don't wear suntan lotion to protect yourself from it. You perceive the results of these energies (for instance, a television program or sunburn) and therefore you trust that they exist. The same is true of healing energy. If you open your mind to the possibility that healing energy exists, you will begin to perceive it.

Everyone is instinctively able to perceive subtle energies without thinking about it. Have you ever walked into a room and noticed a distinct "atmosphere"? If you have, you will have perceived the negative side of healing energy (called disharmonious energy). Have you ever felt great joy in your life, perhaps at achieving a long-held goal, watching your favorite sports team winning the cup or attending a celebration of some sort? Have you ever felt love or loved? If you have, you will have perceived the positive side of healing energy (called harmonious energy). So you see, you *can* perceive healing energy – you just may not have realized it.

The need for balance

Nature is the great rebalancer. No matter what happens in the world, nature always tries to restore itself to a state of balance and harmony. Visit any disused quarry, or the site of a former forest fire, and you will see nature reclaiming the land and restoring the balance. So it is within each one of us. We are part of nature and therefore we need to seek balance and harmony in our lives if we are to become happy and fulfilled. The more we understand our own nature, and the more we discover about different ways of looking at ill health, the better equipped we will become to maintain balance and harmony in our own lives. It will only be through the integration of our scientific understanding in the West with the spiritual understanding of the East that we will be able to fully understand the nature of disease and the solutions to our illnesses. The Western and Eastern concepts of health and healing are not opposite, but complementary and it is this realization that will lead us toward the eradication of illness and disease. It is only through cooperation and integration that mankind will be saved from the path to self-destruction that we are currently on.

RIGHT Visualizing a scene of natural beauty acts as an antidote to the stresses of modern life by calming the mind. Relaxation therapists often use this technique to slow the thought processes and reenergize the body, creating a balance between the mental and the physical.

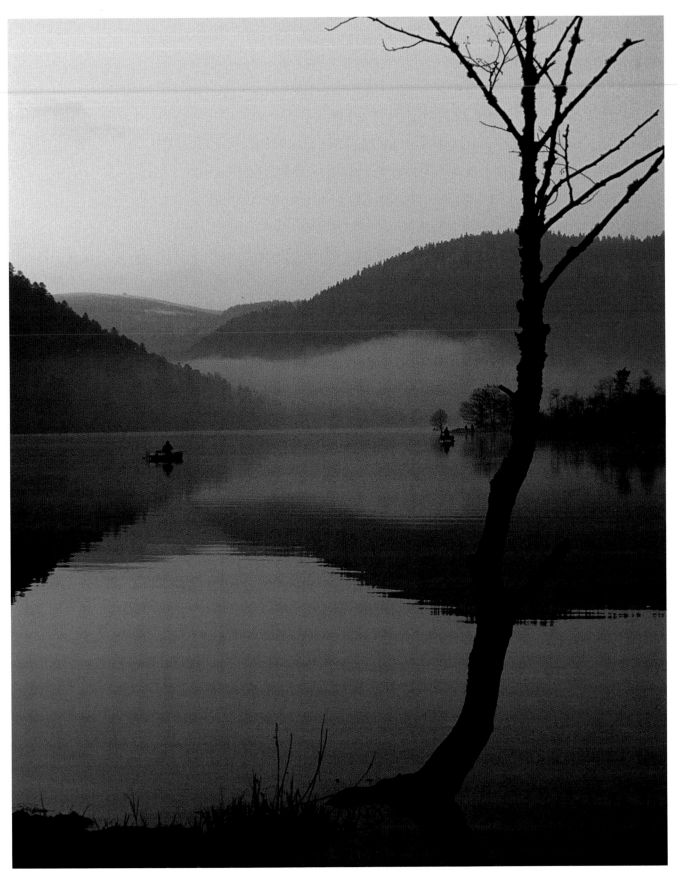

Western and Eastern concepts of health

In its infancy Western medicine promised the almost total eradication of disease. At the beginning of the industrial and scientific revolutions, mankind was given the impression that this explosion of knowledge would make the world a better place for everyone. What has actually happened is that world poverty has increased and more and more people are suffering from more and more illnesses. Certain cancers are dramatically on the increase, as are illnesses such as asthma, eczema, ME (myalgic encephalomyelitis), multiple sclerosis, and arthritis, to name but a few.

Each year we are promised that research is on the brink of amazing new cures, and yet no sooner do we seem to find the solution to one disease than a new strain or variety of illness appears to take its place. When tuberculosis was rife, nobody died from asthma. Now that tuberculosis has been eradicated, thousands of people each year die from asthma and various other lung diseases. Perhaps Western medicine doesn't have all the answers. Perhaps we need to look toward the East, to medical practices that predate our medicine by thousands of years.

Why do we get sick?

Modern medicine tells us that such things as bacteria, viruses and fungi cause many of our illnesses. The causes of many other illnesses such as cancer and ME remain elusive and as a result incurable using Western methods. The Eastern tradition looks at illness in a completely different way, a way which makes the word "incurable" obsolete. It views illness as your body's way of telling you that you are doing something "wrong." Illness is your body posing a question for which you have to find the answer. This means that if you find out what you are doing "wrong" in your life and correct it, there is no need for your body to manifest that illness any more. If this is the

LEFT The driving force behind Western medicine is the search for a cure. Practitioners concentrate on physical symptoms, and though these play a vital role in diagnosing illness, the system ignores the role of the mind which is so important to the Eastern physician.

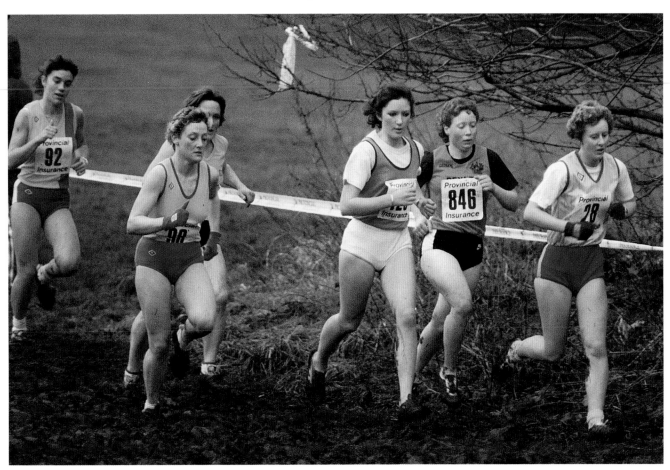

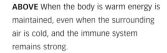

case, it also means that any illness is potentially curable. Let us look at an example.

Western medicine says that a virus causes the common cold. This may be true but why in a class of 20 students who are all exposed to the virus, do some get colds and others not? Clearly the students who do not catch a cold are doing something "right" that the students who do catch a cold are not. Eastern medicine tells us that the common cold is caused by "wind" and "cold" invading the lungs, i.e. the virus attacks those who have allowed the wind and the cold to invade their bodies.

This phenomenon is clearly seen when looking at weekend sports events played in communities throughout the world. The sports players, who wear very little in the way of clothing (often only shorts and a T-shirt) do not catch colds because they are on the move (avoiding the invading "wind") and keeping

warm (avoiding the invading "cold"). The spectators, on the other hand, wearing thick coats and woolens are usually relatively static and, if they are not in prime health, are far more likely to catch a cold. The "wind" and the "cold" are presented with static, easy targets. So in some ways, the common cold is your body's way of telling you to look after yourself better or in a different way.

ABOVE When the body is warm energy is maintained, even when the surrounding air is cold, and the immune system remains strong.

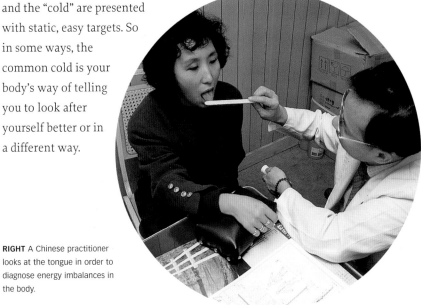

RIGHT A Chinese practitioner looks at the tongue in order to diagnose energy imbalances in the body.

concepts of energy in healing

Western medicine, in its early years, did much of its research by dissecting and studying dead bodies. Obviously a dead body lacks life force and so the concept of energy in healing was ignored. Bodies were regarded as purely mechanical bio-machines that had a tendency to malfunction, rather than unique and complex energy transmitters and receivers whose delicate equilibrium can become upset by discord and disharmony. Oriental medicine, on the other hand, did much of its early research on live bodies and so the concept of energy in healing became fundamental to their medical view.

Western medicine views many illnesses as random occurrences. The victims of "incurable" diseases are powerless pawns of fate. They are just "unlucky." There is an alternative view though. If we take the concept that illness is a message from our bodies to our minds, a question waiting to be answered, then it means that you can potentially find a solution to any illness.

Personal responsibility

Life is a journey filled with opportunities to learn. Illness is just another one of those opportunities. We attract illness to ourselves, not because we are bad, but because we are learners, who can, if we choose, become wise. Illness teaches us to seek more balance and harmony in our lives. If you learn to take responsibility for your illness by acknowledging that it is actually a wonderful opportunity to become a wiser and better person and not some terrible form of

divine punishment, it means that you are no longer a victim. You hold the key to unlocking the doorway to health and fulfillment.

The definition of health

Health is an absence of symptoms according to Western medicine. This is radically different from the Eastern approach. In China, at one time, you paid your "doctor" while you were well. The moment you became ill, you stopped paying and did not start again until total health had been restored. How much healthier we would be if Western medicine adopted the same ethic. Health is much more than an absence of symptoms. It is a state of harmony and balance when an individual feels happy, peaceful, and totally fulfilled with no physical,

LEFT In acupuncture, the insertion of fine needles along the body's energy pathways, or meridians, stimulates the transmission of energy.

emotional, or spiritual illness of any kind. By that definition there are very few truly healthy individuals on the planet, but total health can be the goal – it is the birthright of every individual on the planet.

Claiming health

You have the right to be healthy and fulfilled. Just because you are not totally healthy and balanced does not mean that you abandon that right. On the contrary, it means that you search even more diligently for the answers to the questions your body is giving you. You have the ability within you to find those answers. You have many powers that can be unlocked to help you find your goal and intuition is perhaps the chief of these powers. Every individual possesses it and it is intuition that will show you the way ahead.

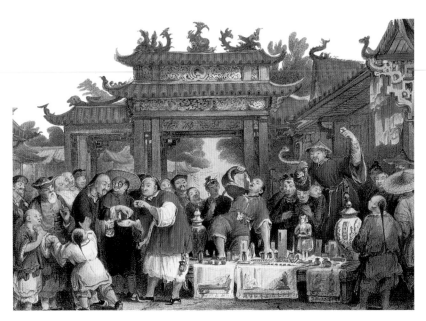

BELOW While medieval physicians in the West were dissecting bodies to find out how they worked, the Chinese were rewriting the Nei-Ching, a classic medical treatise first compiled between 400 and 250 B.C.E.

ABOVE Chinese medicine is one of the oldest systems in the world. A Chinese doctor attracts a crowd in this engraving of 1843.

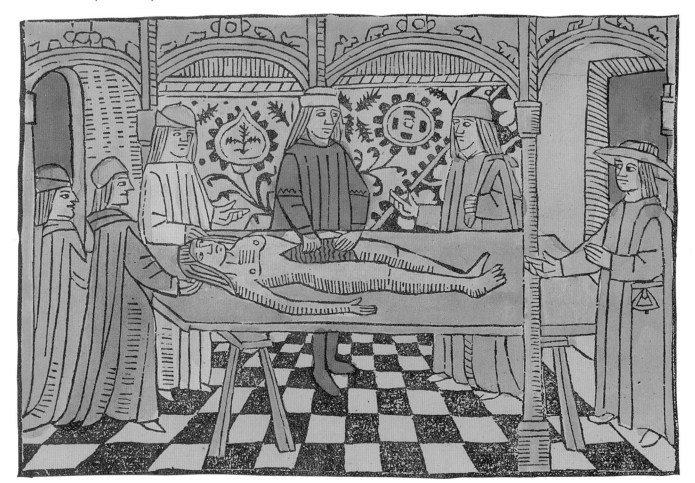

using intuition

Intuition is one of the body's ways of perceiving the paths to solutions. It is that part of you that tells you if you are right or wrong. It is a part of our being that we fail to use efficiently because we do not use it regularly. Everything you come across in life needs to be tested and the best test is with the intuition. Take the first sentence of this paragraph: does it ring true with you, do you think it is wrong or do you not know? When you test how something "feels" you are using your intuition and from the feedback you get from your intuition, you make a judgement. Judgements are not fixed in stone; they are merely how you perceive something at that time. For instance, you may judge the sentence at the beginning of the paragraph to be wrong, only to discover later that you were mistaken. This is intuition working at its best.

The sense of intuition is never wrong, though occasionally we perceive it incorrectly. Usually if your intuition leads you to reject something that you later find out to be true, it is just your intuition telling you that you were not ready to learn that lesson at the time you rejected it. There are never mistakes, only lessons waiting to be learned. Our intuition guides us on our journey of learning and if we maintain an attitude of healthy curiosity, it will guide us to all the answers we seek.

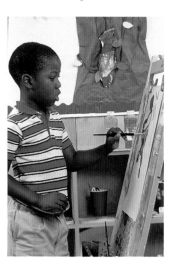

LEFT Children's natural curiosity and willingness to learn are the foundations of their intuition.

RIGHT Develop your intuition by listening or "tuning in" to it when making decisions.

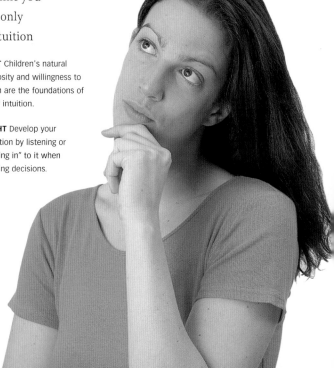

Eastern philosophy teaches that energy is moved by the mind. This means that every thought-form is energy and that by harnessing the energy of those thoughts, we can control our destinies. You are what you think. To prove this concept of the mind moving your energy, you can conduct two experiments to show how your mind can control your energy. You will need a friend to help you conduct them.

Experiment 1

Stand about 3 feet (1m) away from a wall and get a friend to stand next you on your right-hand side and facing you. Bend your right elbow and point your forearm and fist toward the wall. Now get your partner to place his/her left hand on your elbow and their right hand on your wrist. Get your partner to try to force your

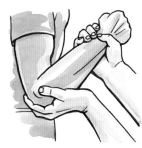

STEP 3 Ask your partner to force your hand up toward your shoulder. Using muscle power try to resist – you will probably find that your partner has the upper hand.

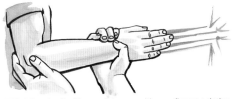

STEP 4 Now try it with your fist open with your fingers pointing toward the wall. Visualize red paint shooting out of your fingers and hitting the wall. You will find that resistance is easier.

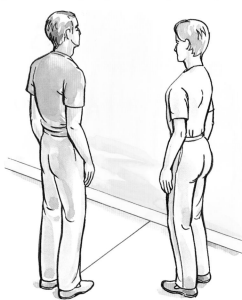

STEP 1 Stand about 3 feet (1m) away from a wall with a partner standing next to you, then bend your right elbow and point your forearm and fist toward the wall.

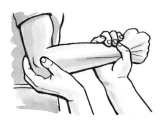

STEP 2 Ask your partner to place their left hand on your elbow and their right hand on your wrist.

hand up toward your shoulder while you try to resist using muscle power. If you are evenly matched in strength, you will probably lose.

Try the experiment again, but this time open your fist, point your fingers toward the wall and imagine red paint shooting out of your fingers and hitting the wall. Don't use muscle power, just keep thinking of the red paint. You should now find it easy to resist your partner no matter how strong they are. This is because you are using your mind to direct your energy, and your energy is much stronger than your muscles. The image of red paint is used here as a strong image that is easy for most people to visualize. You could use any strong image. Try visualizing white light or a different colored paint and see if it makes any difference.

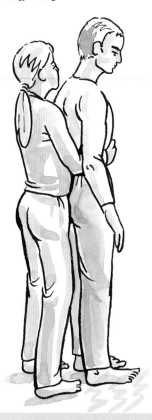

Experiment 2

Ask your partner to stand behind you. They are going to put their arms around your waist and try to pick you up twice. The first time, think light, airy thoughts. Visualize energy flowing out of the top of your head and think of yourself as light as a feather. Your partner should find it easy to pick you up.

The second time project all of your energy down through your feet. Imagine roots growing out of your feet and into the ground. Think yourself heavy. Your partner should now find it much harder to pick you up despite the fact that your actual weight will not have changed. The only difference between the two lifts is how you manipulate your own energy with your thoughts.

SENSING ENERGY

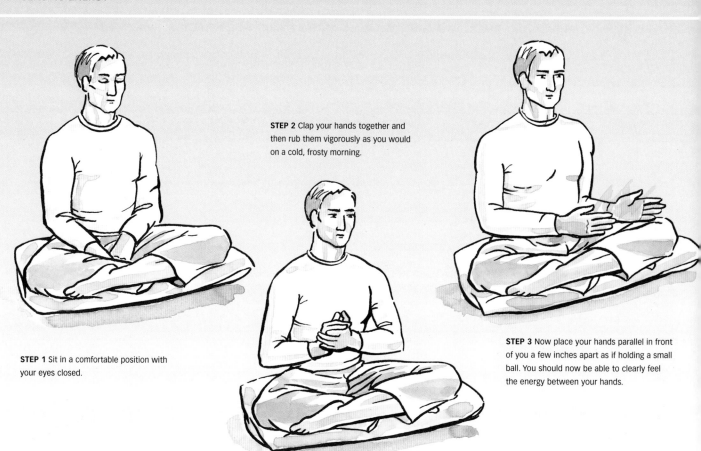

STEP 1 Sit in a comfortable position with your eyes closed.

STEP 2 Clap your hands together and then rub them vigorously as you would on a cold, frosty morning.

STEP 3 Now place your hands parallel in front of you a few inches apart as if holding a small ball. You should now be able to clearly feel the energy between your hands.

The five spiritual aspects

Traditional Chinese medicine recognizes five spiritual aspects of life: shen, chen, hun, po, and I (the sum total of the other four aspects). All of the five aspects need to be in balance and harmony for an individual to be healthy. Shen is best described as a feeling of upliftedness or joy in one's life – a time to be happy, relaxed, and free of worry. Chen is associated with strength and determination and the ability to achieve things – a time to undertake work. Po is a sense of social belonging and interaction, for it is only through our interaction with others that we can truly improve ourselves – a time for others. Hun is a sense of destiny and purpose – a time to concentrate upon the self.

If your "I" can display all four aspects of shen, chen, po and hun in balance then the chances are that you will be a healthy individual. We know that all work (chen) and no play (shen) "makes Jack a dull boy," but equally all play and no work can cause a lack of focus in your life that will eventually lead to a sense of powerlessness. Everyone needs to find time for self-expression (hun) and time to interact and learn from other people (po). Those who shun any contact with the rest of society can become very sad and lonely people. Equally those who are totally selfless do not find the path to happiness. Follow the Chinese principle of constantly seeking a balance of all four aspects in your life and you will be on the road to health and happiness.

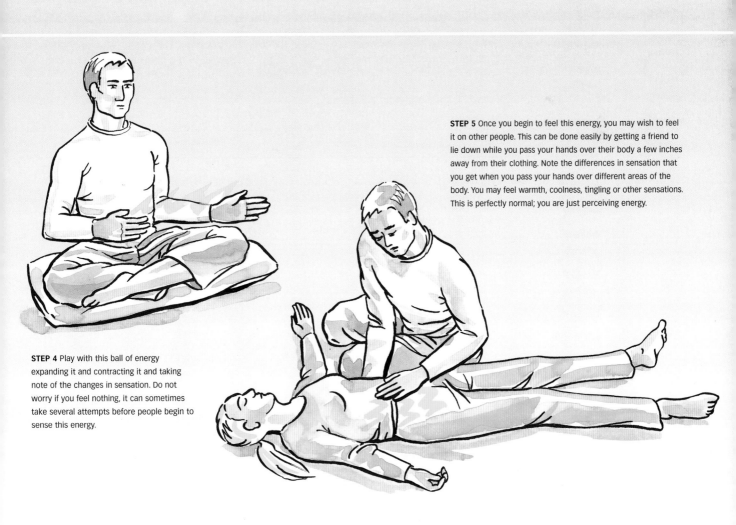

STEP 5 Once you begin to feel this energy, you may wish to feel it on other people. This can be done easily by getting a friend to lie down while you pass your hands over their body a few inches away from their clothing. Note the differences in sensation that you get when you pass your hands over different areas of the body. You may feel warmth, coolness, tingling or other sensations. This is perfectly normal; you are just perceiving energy.

STEP 4 Play with this ball of energy expanding it and contracting it and taking note of the changes in sensation. Do not worry if you feel nothing, it can sometimes take several attempts before people begin to sense this energy.

Modern science meets ancient wisdom

Until recently, the gap between alternative therapies and Western medicine has been huge, but this is now changing due to modern science. Scientists have been conducting clinical trials in China, Japan, and the West to try to prove the validity of many alternative therapies with encouraging results. Some things at present defy scientific explanation but, with the advances that science is making, it is only a matter of time before science "catches up" with ancient wisdom.

One of the most amazing documented uses of Western medicine meeting alternative therapies is in the use of acupuncture and hypnotism in place of traditional anesthesia in major operations. Operations that have been carried out using acupuncture or hypnosis instead of anesthetic drugs include tooth extraction, removal of cataracts, tonsillectomy, thyroidectomy, hernia repair, bone fracture repair, open heart surgery, and stomach surgery.

Acupuncture anaesthesia involves giving pain relief to a patient during a surgical procedure by merely inserting acupuncture needles in certain specific points. The patient remains conscious throughout the procedure, allowing them to cooperate fully with the surgeon. This is of particular use when surgery involves the brain. The patient under acupuncture anesthesia has clear mental function, speech, sensations, and limb movements that can provide instant feedback to the surgeon and thus avert accidental damage to the sensory, motor, or cranial nerves during surgery. Patients also recover more quickly because they suffer no side effects from drugs. Obviously an anesthetist is always on hand "just in case" but they are not called on in the majority of circumstances. The method is simple, practical, and economical, and may, one day, be the standard practice in most surgery.

RIGHT The body has 14 main meridians, or energy pathways. Modern acupuncture uses points along these pathways to treat illness.

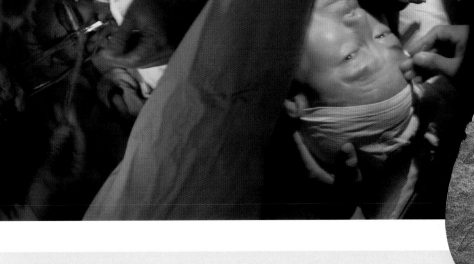

LEFT Acupuncture is used as an anesthetic during a lung operation in Shanghai.

CANCER AND CHI KUNG

Many studies of alternative therapies have revolved around the treatment of cancer. Chi kung is one such therapy that has achieved encouraging results in China with cancer patients. For example, a study by Sun Qui-zhi and Zhao Li of the Kuangan Men Hospital in China looked at the effectiveness of Chi kung on patients suffering from advanced, medically diagnosed, malignant cancer with the following results:

	Control group (Taking drugs only)	**Chi kung group** (Combining drugs and Chi Kung)
No of patients	102	102
Dosage of drug	"regular"	"small"
Results after 6 months:		
Blood viscosity	no improvement	improved
Platelet abnormalities	no improvement	improved
Results after 6 years:		
Clinical effectiveness	68%(+or- 1%)	87%(+or-3%)
Total mortality	32.0%	17.3%

This is just one of the hundreds of studies now being carried out which will one day help to bridge the gap between the East and West.

RIGHT Chi kung is a gentle exercise system developed in China. Tai chi is sometimes called moving chi kung.

Yin and yang

According to ancient Chinese myth, before the world we now live in was created there was nothing but chaos. This time is known as Wu-Chi and can be described as a state of "disorganized formlessness." Out of this chaos was born tai chi. The tai chi symbol is a pictorial representation of the workings of the universe and of the dynamic interaction between two forces called yin and yang.

Yin and yang are opposites, but they are also complementary. They are two forces that can be used to describe anything in the universe because everything in the universe is made up of two parts in a state of dynamic equilibrium with one another. The cycle of a day is made up of light and dark, molecules are made up of positively and negatively charged molecules, and even men and women bear some physical aspects of their opposite sex. Everything is made up of yin and yang qualities. Yin and yang provide us with many

THE CHARACTERISTICS OF YIN AND YANG

1 Everything that exists can be described in terms of two opposite and complementary forces (yin and yang).

2 Yin is centrifugal, expansive, and cooling. Yang is centripetal, compacting and warming.

3 Yin attracts yang and yang attracts yin (i.e. this attraction is seen between male and female and between positive and negative ions).

4 All that exists is composed of yin and yang in different proportions.

5 Nothing is completely yin or completely yang (there are no true absolutes in the universe).

6 Yin and yang are never static, but always in the state of dynamic movement (just as night gives way to day and vice versa).

7 In all that exists there is always either yin or yang in excess (nothing in the universe is truly neutral).

8 Yin repels yin and yang repels yang ("like repels like" is a fundamental law of ionic chemistry).

9 Yin produces yang and yang produces yin (heat produces fire, fire produces steam etc.).

BELOW Trigrams made up of broken and unbroken lines symbolize yin and yang.

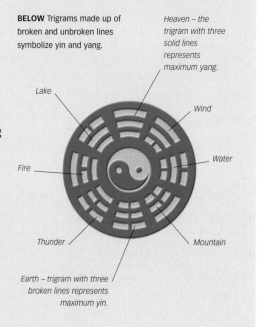

Heaven – the trigram with three solid lines represents maximum yang.

Lake

Wind

Fire

Water

Thunder

Mountain

Earth – trigram with three broken lines represents maximum yin.

YIN AND YANG CLASSIFICATIONS OF FOOD

THE TABLE MOVES FROM YIN TO YANG VERTICALLY

OILS	DRINKS	FRUITS	DAIRY	VEG	CEREALS	FISH	ANIMAL	OTHERS
Coconut oil**	Artificially sweet	Pineapple	Yogurt***	Eggplant	Corn*	Oyster*	Snail**	Sugar***
Peanut oil	Dyed tea***	Mango***	Sour cream	Tomato***	Rye	Clam	Frog	Honey
Olive oil	Coffee	Grapefruit	Cream	Potato	Barley	Octopus	Pork	Molasses
Soybean oil	Fruit juice	Banana	Cream cheese	Shiitake	Oats	Carp	Beef	Fructose
Sunflower oil*	Champagne	Fig	Butter	Beans+	Wheat	Mussels	Horsemeat	Rice syrup**
Corn oil	Wine	Orange	Cow's milk**	Cucumber	Rice**	Halibut	Hare	
Sesame oil	Beer**	Pear	Camembert	Spinach	Millet	Lobster	Chicken*	
Safflower oil	Mineral water	Peach**	Gruyère	Asparagus	Buckwheat@@	Trout	Pigeon@	
	Carbonated water	Lime	Roquefort@	Artichoke		Sole	Duck	
	Water	Melon	Edam	Mushroom		Salmon@	Turkey	
	Bancha tea*	Almond	Goat's milk@@	Peas**		Shrimp	Eggs@@	
	Yannoh	Peanut	Goat's cheese	Celery		Herring	Pheasant@@@	
	Mu tea@@	Cashew		Cauliflower		Sardine		
	Ginseng@@@	Filbert		Broccoli		Red snapper		
		Olive*		Purple cabbage		Caviar@@		
		Cherry		Beet				
		Strawberry@		Green cabbage				
		Chestnut		Lettuce@				
		Apple@@		Endive				
				Kale				
				Turnip				
				Radish				
				Onion				
				Pumpkin@@				
				Carrot				
				Watercress				

*** VERY YIN   ** MORE YIN   * YIN   @@@ VERY YANG   @@ MORE YANG   @ YANG   +Except Adzuki

ways of comparing things. When comparing something that is hot with something that is cold, heat is described as yang and cold as yin. When comparing something that is hot with something that is hotter, heat is described as yin and extreme heat is described as yang. So everything that is hot is not necessary yang; it depends what you are comparing it with. You can only compare one aspect at a time when describing things in terms of the yin and yang. For instance, traditionally yin represents the feminine and coolness while yang represents the masculine and warmth, but try to compare a cold man to warm woman in terms of yin and yang and you will get into great difficulties.

TRADITIONAL ATTRIBUTES GIVEN TO YIN AND YANG

YIN	YANG
Masculine	Feminine
Death	Birth
Purple	Scarlet
Night	Day
Dark	Light
Cold	Hot
Acid	Alkaline
Potassium	Sodium
Expansive, light	Contractile, dense

The five elements

From yin and yang, the ancient Chinese developed the theory of the five elements or breaths (Wu-Hsing) and they used these five elements to describe the cyclic nature of the universe. The five elements are translated as wood, fire, earth, metal, and water. The laws of the physical universe cause these elements to interact with one another endlessly (see chart opposite). For instance:

A tree (wood) when burned (fire) produces steam (water) and ash (earth). The ash is compacted over millions of years to form ores (metal).

Wood creates fire (rubbing two sticks together), but water destroys fire. A stone (earth) blunts or sharpens an ax (metal) depending on how it is used.

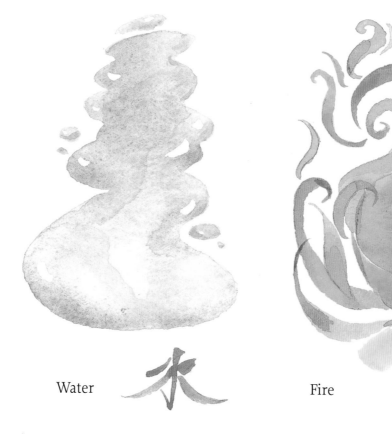

Water   水   Fire   火

THE QUALITIES OF THE FIVE ELEMENTS AND THEIR ASSOCIATION WITH THE BODY

Element	Wood	Fire	Earth	Metal	Water
Direction	East	South	Center	West	North
Season	Spring	Summer	Indian summer	Autumn	Winter
Climate	Windy	Hot	Damp	Dry	Cold
Emotion	Anger	Joy	Pensive	Grief	Fear
Taste	Sour	Bitter	Sweet	Pungent	Salty
Sense organ	Eye	Tongue	Mouth	Nose	Ear
Yin organ	Liver	Heart	Spleen	Lungs	Kidney
Yang organ	Gallbladder	Small intestine	Stomach	Large intestine	Urinary bladder
Tissue	Tendons	Blood vessels	Flesh	Skin	Bones
Western element	Fire	Water	Ether	Air	Earth

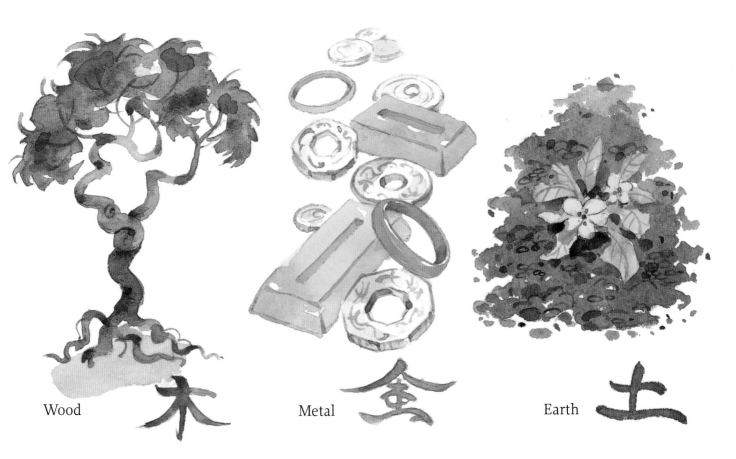

Wood   Metal   Earth

2 body energetics

For thousands of years the cultures of the East have known about the existence of special energies that run throughout and around the body. In China they call this energy "chi," in Japan "ki," and in India "prana." In the physical world we cannot see the subtle energies of radio waves and microwaves but they do exist. So it is with our bodies: there are many subtle energies around and throughout our bodies that we cannot physically see but which do exist. Just as we can confirm that radio waves exist through our experience of listening to the radio, so too there are ways in which we can perceive the subtle energies of the body. This can be done by touch, by dowsing, and a whole host of other methods.

The aura

Around every living thing is a collection of electromagnetic energies vibrating at different densities. They are held around the body by electromagnetic attraction and form an oval shape called the "auric egg." This energy field, called the aura, extends outside of the physical body an average of 3 feet (1m) and is layered like an onion. Plants, animals, and even crystals all have their own unique auras. There are some people who have the ability to see auras very clearly and they often describe them as beautiful, multicolored bands of light.

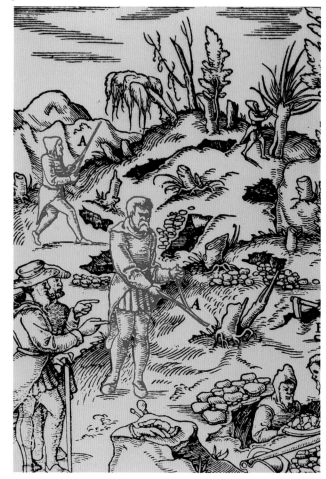

RIGHT Dowsing was once used to locate underground metal for mining, as shown in this illustration from *De Re Metallica*, written by German metallurgist Georgius Agricola in 1555.

LEARNING TO SEE AURAS

It is not only gifted psychics who can see auras, anyone can with the proper training. Auras are seen using our peripheral vision, using those receptors in our eyes that see low-light images. Learning to focus your mind on the following low-light receptors will enable you to start to see auras:

1 In a low-lit room, find a dark, plain background (a piece of dark cloth, curtain, or wallpaper).

2 Place your hand a few inches (centimeters) above the cloth with your fingers spread.

3 Take a few moments to "tune in" by focusing your mind on the fact that you want to see auras and take a few deep, slow breaths to help you to relax.

4 Stare at your hand with a relaxed, unfocused stare, trying to not let your eyes focus on any one point but to take in the whole picture.

5 Without changing your focus, bring your mind's attention to the area between your fingers. If you concentrate, you will begin to see a hazy glow around the fingers.

6 Introduce the other hand to your field of vision and see if you can perceive the energy between your hands, which you felt in the sensing energy exercise on page 18.

7 Now place your open palms so that your fingertips are only a few inches (centimeters) apart and see if you can perceive strands of energy connecting your fingers that move and bend as you move your hands.

Do not worry if you do not succeed in seeing auras first time. Keep practicing and you will succeed. Once you have mastered the technique of seeing your own aura, you can try to see the auras in normal light or look at the auras of plants, animals, or crystals.

RIGHT Detecting auras takes concentration and practice, and the willingness to tune into a universal spiritual energy.

Subtle body energies

The physical body is not the only body that we possess. The energies that make up the aura are called subtle bodies comprising the etheric body, the astral/emotional body, the mental body, and the spiritual body. These subtle bodies are made of pure energy, with each body vibrating at a progressively higher vibrational rate.

The table below demonstrates the rate at which each of these subtle bodies vibrates. The etheric body vibrates at the slowest rate and the spiritual body at the highest rate. The subtle bodies are also interpenetrating, with the etheric body interpenetrating the

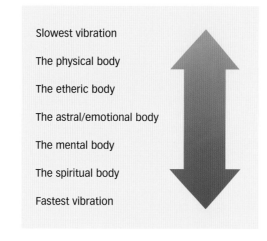

Slowest vibration

The physical body

The etheric body

The astral/emotional body

The mental body

The spiritual body

Fastest vibration

physical body; the astral body interpenetrating the etheric and the physical bodies; the mental body interpenetrating the astral, etheric, and physical bodies; and the spiritual body interpenetrating each of the other four subtle bodies.

The physical body

This is the body that we know best. It is the one we use to express our lives with. It is the one that manifests illness, but often the imbalance begins in the subtle bodies.

The etheric body

In terms of energy healing, the etheric body is perhaps the most important. It is a perfect blueprint of the physical body, which it is connected to and helps to maintain. It is usually seen a few inches (centimeters) outside the physical body following its outline. It acts as a transformer of subtle energies (such as those emanating from a healing crystal), allowing them to enter the body via the central nervous system and the endocrine (glandular) and circulatory systems. When perfectly aligned with the physical body, it facilitates clear access to the path of destiny. It is also the body that facilitates the transmission and receipt of telepathic messages.

The etheric body holds a perfect blueprint of the physical body and it is thought that energy imbalances in the etheric bodies of amputees may be the cause of phantom pain in amputated limbs. It is also the body that makes the occasionally reported regrowing of such things as severed fingers or new eyes possible – things that are labelled "beyond belief" or "miraculous."

Those with the ability to see this body, see a white glow around the physical body in a healthy individual; those who have stronger abilities, see a beautifully colored rainbow beginning with red below the feet and changing through orange and yellow as it

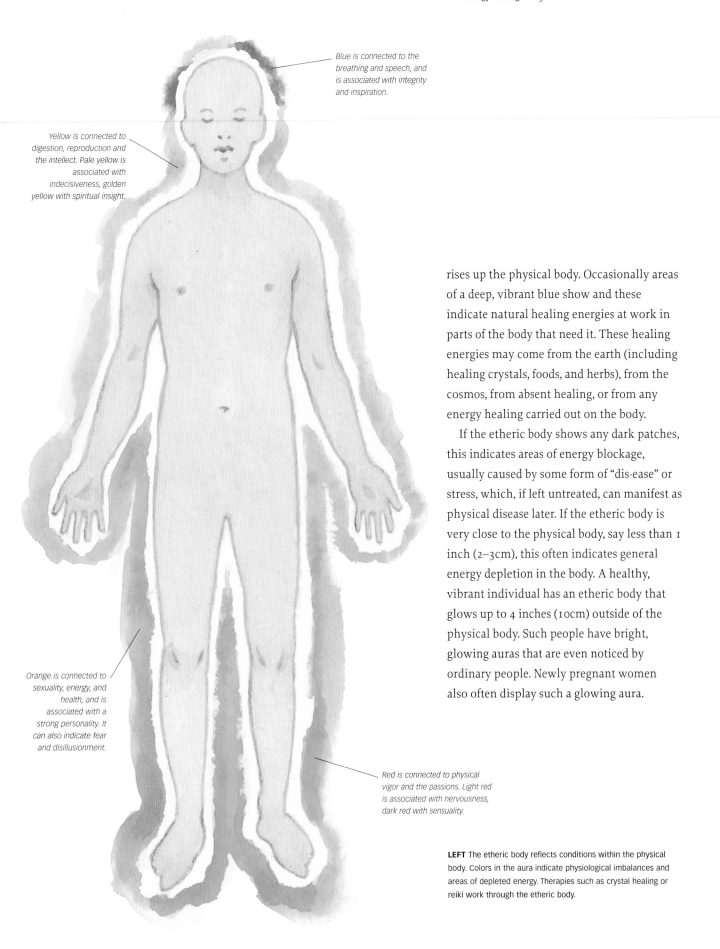

Blue is connected to the breathing and speech, and is associated with integrity and inspiration.

Yellow is connected to digestion, reproduction and the intellect. Pale yellow is associated with indecisiveness, golden yellow with spiritual insight.

Orange is connected to sexuality, energy, and health, and is associated with a strong personality. It can also indicate fear and disillusionment.

Red is connected to physical vigor and the passions. Light red is associated with nervousness, dark red with sensuality.

rises up the physical body. Occasionally areas of a deep, vibrant blue show and these indicate natural healing energies at work in parts of the body that need it. These healing energies may come from the earth (including healing crystals, foods, and herbs), from the cosmos, from absent healing, or from any energy healing carried out on the body.

If the etheric body shows any dark patches, this indicates areas of energy blockage, usually caused by some form of "dis-ease" or stress, which, if left untreated, can manifest as physical disease later. If the etheric body is very close to the physical body, say less than 1 inch (2–3cm), this often indicates general energy depletion in the body. A healthy, vibrant individual has an etheric body that glows up to 4 inches (10cm) outside of the physical body. Such people have bright, glowing auras that are even noticed by ordinary people. Newly pregnant women also often display such a glowing aura.

LEFT The etheric body reflects conditions within the physical body. Colors in the aura indicate physiological imbalances and areas of depleted energy. Therapies such as crystal healing or reiki work through the etheric body.

The astral/emotional body

The astral body forms an oval around and beyond the etheric and the physical bodies and is usually perceived as varying shades of green. It is also called the emotional body because it is in full activity when we are aroused, excited, frightened or in any way emotionally charged. These feelings are often "divorced" from the rational mind and can lead to great imbalance. Western scientists and doctors are now beginning to realize that emotions play a vital role in the health of an individual. Negative emotions such as hatred, anger, resentment, and jealousy cause disharmony and imbalance in the astral body which in turn can manifest in the etheric and physical bodies as "dis-ease" and disease respectively. Positive emotions such as love, joy, and positivity can equally have a beneficial effect on an imbalanced etheric or physical body and greatly speed up the healing process.

A clear, green astral body indicates a healthy individual who is in touch with their own emotions while at the same time being aware and considerate of the emotions of others. A dull green color is often indicative of someone who has been emotionally drained by those around them, while a yellow-green color can indicate jealousy and resentment, which tend to interrupt the free flow of energy around the astral body. Dark areas indicate unresolved pain and hurt stored in the astral body, and areas devoid of color often indicate unresolved guilt.

The astral body is at its most active when two people feel a strong emotion between them such as love or dislike. When two people feel love, their astral bodies vibrate harmoniously and interlink. This is why two people in love still feel a strong emotional bond even when apart. Dislike between two individuals manifests in their astral bodies as a discordant clash, which can cause damage to both parties if unresolved.

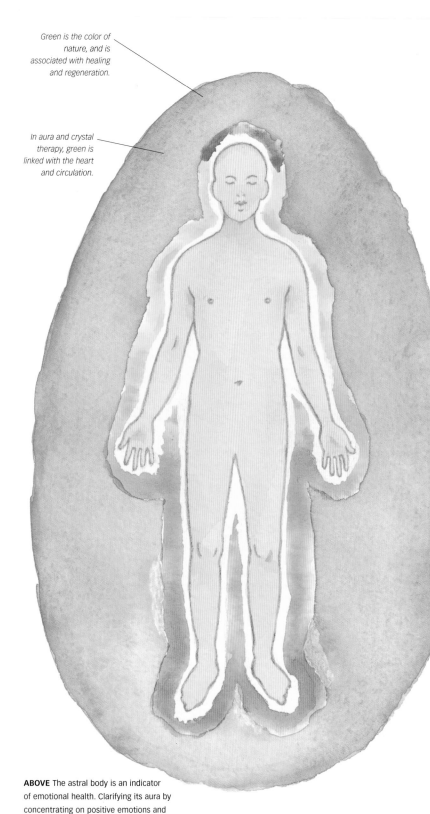

Green is the color of nature, and is associated with healing and regeneration.

In aura and crystal therapy, green is linked with the heart and circulation.

ABOVE The astral body is an indicator of emotional health. Clarifying its aura by concentrating on positive emotions and resolving painful or stressful issues helps to heal the physical body.

Violet and gold are the colors of spiritual enlightenment.

The mental body

This body forms an outer layer around the astral body and is the same oval shape. It is colored blue, turning to purple as it rises up the body. In spiritually evolved individuals, this body is colored white, silver, or gold above and around the head, depicted as a halo in medieval art. In a mentally unstable or depressed person, the area above and around the head can be seen as gray, brown, or black. This body is most active when our thoughts are clear and our intent pure.

The spiritual body

This body is usually colored white with shades of purple, gold, or silver. It is the body that connects us to the cosmos and to our higher spiritual selves. In powerful shamans and healers, this body can extend several feet (meters) outside the physical body.

White patches in the outer subtle bodies indicate spiritual attunement.

LEFT The color and tone of the mental body reflects psychological health, and the spiritual body emanates from it. Concentrating the mind through regular meditation can purify these bodies and extend the spiritual aura.

Chakras

Chakras are energy centers in and around the body that can be likened to swirling vortices or whirlpools of energy. The word chakra comes from an ancient Sanskrit word meaning "wheel." Early Tibetan Sanskrit manuscripts spoke of three chakras. This later increased to five and then to seven. Today it is acknowledged that there are other minor chakras in the body in addition to the major seven, and that each swirls at its own speed and frequency of vibration.

The ancients assigned one of each of the colors of the rainbow to each of the seven primary chakras, which were regarded as harmonic resonances of the vibrational frequencies of the individual chakras. This means that if a chakra was perceived as spinning out of balance, or too fast or too slow, introducing a color to the area of the chakra helped to restore its proper spin again, thus in turn restoring health.

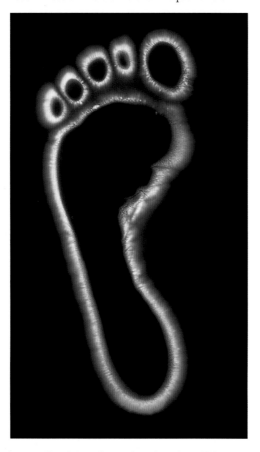

ABOVE Kirlian photographs are taken using a sheet of light-sensitive paper laid on top of a metal plate. A high-voltage current is then passed through the plate. The resulting image shows a luminous elecromagnetic field around the edges of the body.

Measuring aura and chakra energies

In 1869 the English physician and surgeon, Walter John Kilner, was appointed as head of one of the world's first X ray departments at St. Thomas' Hospital, London. Kilner became fascinated with attempting to photograph luminous energy emanations of the human body and to this end created a lens coated with a dye called dicyanin. This dye-coated lens allowed one to see light from the ultraviolet range. The whole apparatus, which become known as a Kilner screen, made it possible to see one or two bands of blue-gray light, which extended about 15–20 cm (6–8 inches) around the outside of the body.

In the 1930s and 1940s, the Russian scientist Semyon Kirlian, invented a special technique for reproducing an image of the emanations of the body on photographic paper. Kirlian photography is now used as a diagnostic technique by some energy healers and other alternative practitioners.

THE SEVEN MAJOR CHAKRAS

The seven chakras are acknowledged by many complementary therapies, and their imbalances can be diagnosed or treated using crystals, dowsing, flower essences, polarity therapy, or visualization techniques.

THE SEVENTH/CROWN CHAKRA: located at the crown of the head and denoted by the color violet, this chakra is the center of spirituality and enlightenment. It vitalizes the cerebrum and the pineal gland.

THE SIXTH/THIRD-EYE/BROW CHAKRA: located between the eyebrows and denoted by the color indigo, this chakra is the center of psychic power and higher intuition. It vitalizes the eyes, cerebellum, the central nervous system, and the pituitary gland.

THE FIFTH/THROAT CHAKRA: located at the neck and denoted by the color blue, this chakra is the center of communication and expression. It vitalizes the throat, lungs, vocal chords, and the thyroid gland.

THE FOURTH/HEART CHAKRA: located in the center of the chest and denoted by the color green, this chakra is the center of love. It vitalizes the heart and the thymus gland.

THE THIRD/SOLAR PLEXUS CHAKRA: located just below the sternum (breast bone) and denoted by the color yellow, this chakra is the center of personal power and ambition. It vitalizes the stomach, liver, gallbladder, sympathetic nervous system, pancreas, spleen, and adrenal glands.

THE SECOND/SACRAL CHAKRA: located just below the navel and denoted by the color orange, this chakra is connected to our desires, emotions, creativity, and sexuality. It vitalizes the digestive system and the sexual organs.

THE ROOT/BASE CHAKRA: located at the base of the spine and denoted by the color red, this chakra is connected to physical strength, determination and courage. It vitalizes the kidneys, the suprarenal glands and the spinal column.

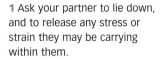

Chakra balancing and healing

There are several simple, yet powerful energy healing techniques to help balance the chakras. The technique below is one of them. However, do not attempt to cleanse, heal, or balance the chakras of another until you have balanced your own chakras. If this is not done, a transfer of imbalance can take place, to the detriment of the one you wish to help. Do not use this technique on children without taking particular care and never above the throat. This is because it is potentially dangerous to try to work on the brow and crown chakras above the throat while any imbalance remains in the lower chakras. Although you should balance your own chakras first, for the purposes of describing this technique it is assumed that you are helping someone else. A pendulum is used as both a diagnostic and healing tool. You can purchase glass, wooden, or crystal pendulums from most New Age outlets or make your own with a ring and a piece of thread.

1 Ask your partner to lie down, and to release any stress or strain they may be carrying within them.

2 Settle yourself down comfortably beside them and take a few slow, deep breaths.

3 Visualize roots growing down from your body to connect you to the earth and strands of white light connecting you to the Divine. Remember that you are acting only as a channel for healing energies and that your intention should be one of pure harmony and love.

4 Hold your pendulum still over the base chakra and watch it to pick up the spin of the chakra.

5 Ask that it be cleansed, harmonized, balanced, and aligned. As you do this, the spin continues.

6 When the process is finished, the pendulum becomes still.

7 Repeat this in turn for the sacral, solar plexus, heart, and throat chakras. Do not worry if the pendulum spins in different directions for different chakras. This is perfectly normal. Do not proceed beyond these until you have made the lower chakras clear and balanced.

8 When you have done the throat, move back to the base chakra visualizing the energies of your partner being drawn down to the base, then ask that all chakras be harmonized, balanced, and aligned together.

9 Your pendulum will rotate, then fall still when the process is complete.

10 Finally, visualize both you and your partner being bathed and protected by pure love. Take a few deep breaths, offer thanks in whatever way you wish and finish.

Chinese view of body energy

The Chinese call energy chi or qi. All chi is considered healthy, nourishing energy. Unhealthy energy is called sha.

The different types of energy are as follows:

Jing (essence): This is the energy we inherit from our parents and is our basic life force. It can be added to or depleted, depending on lifestyle and general health. It is stored in the kidneys and controls life cycles, growth, and reproduction.

Yuan chi: This is the energy of our unique genetic blueprint, which acts as a catalyst for jing after birth, stimulating life and growth.

Zhong chi: This is called the energy of the chest and is the energy that allows the heart and lungs to remain healthy.

Zhen chi: This is the basic body energy made from zhong chi catalyzed by yuan chi and is found all over the body as wei chi and ying chi.

Ying chi: This is the energy whose flow starts at the lungs and circulates throughout the body in the meridians (see page 36) and organs.

Wei chi: This is our defensive energy, which flows through our skin and muscles and joins the physical body to the etheric body.

Gu chi: Translated as food essence, this energy is formed from our food by the spleen and rises to the lungs to combine with the energy we extract from the air we breath to form zhong chi.

LEFT Tai chi is a slow, flowing sequence of movements that balance and energize the life force.

BELOW A tai chi master leads a group in a park in Hong Kong. The sequences require many hours of practice but bring many benefits, from healthier bones and internal organs to clarity of mind.

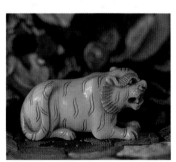

ABOVE In tai chi, the tiger is a symbol of the ego, which is mastered through constant practice.

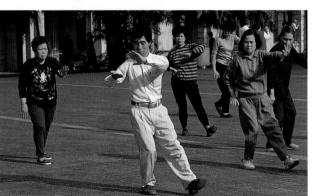

The meridians

Energy travels throughout the body through channels known as meridians. These meridians form an interconnected energy system similar to a telephone system, allowing energy to flow freely to every area of the body. There are 12 regular meridians that correspond to each of the six yin and yang organs in the body. There are also eight extra meridians, but only two of them are considered major meridians. These are the governing vessel and the conception vessel and they connect the back and front of the body, running up the mid-line of the body at the front and down the spine at the back.

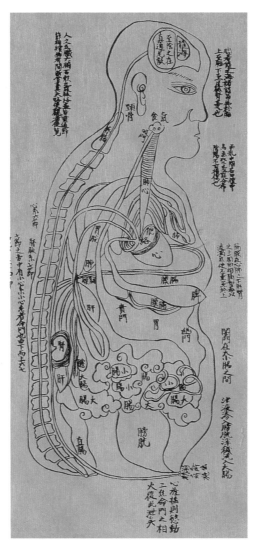

Disharmonies in an organ can make themselves manifest in the corresponding meridian as a blockage or excess of energy. For instance, the liver meridian is connected to the eyes; so an overactive liver may manifest as redness in the eyes. The kidney meridian is connected to the ears; so an over- or under-active kidney may manifest as ear problems.

Yin and yang meridians

The major yin meridians and their corresponding yang meridians are as follows:

The heart: This meridian is the most important meridian since it controls the blood and blood vessels whose proper functioning is essential to life. The meridian opens into the tongue (speech problems are often related to the heart) and its corresponding yang meridian is the small intestine.

The liver: This meridian controls blood storage and maintains the free flow of energy around the body. It also controls the muscles and

LEFT A Chinese acupuncture chart shows the correspondence between the body's energy and its internal organs.

THE MERIDIANS - FRONT VIEW

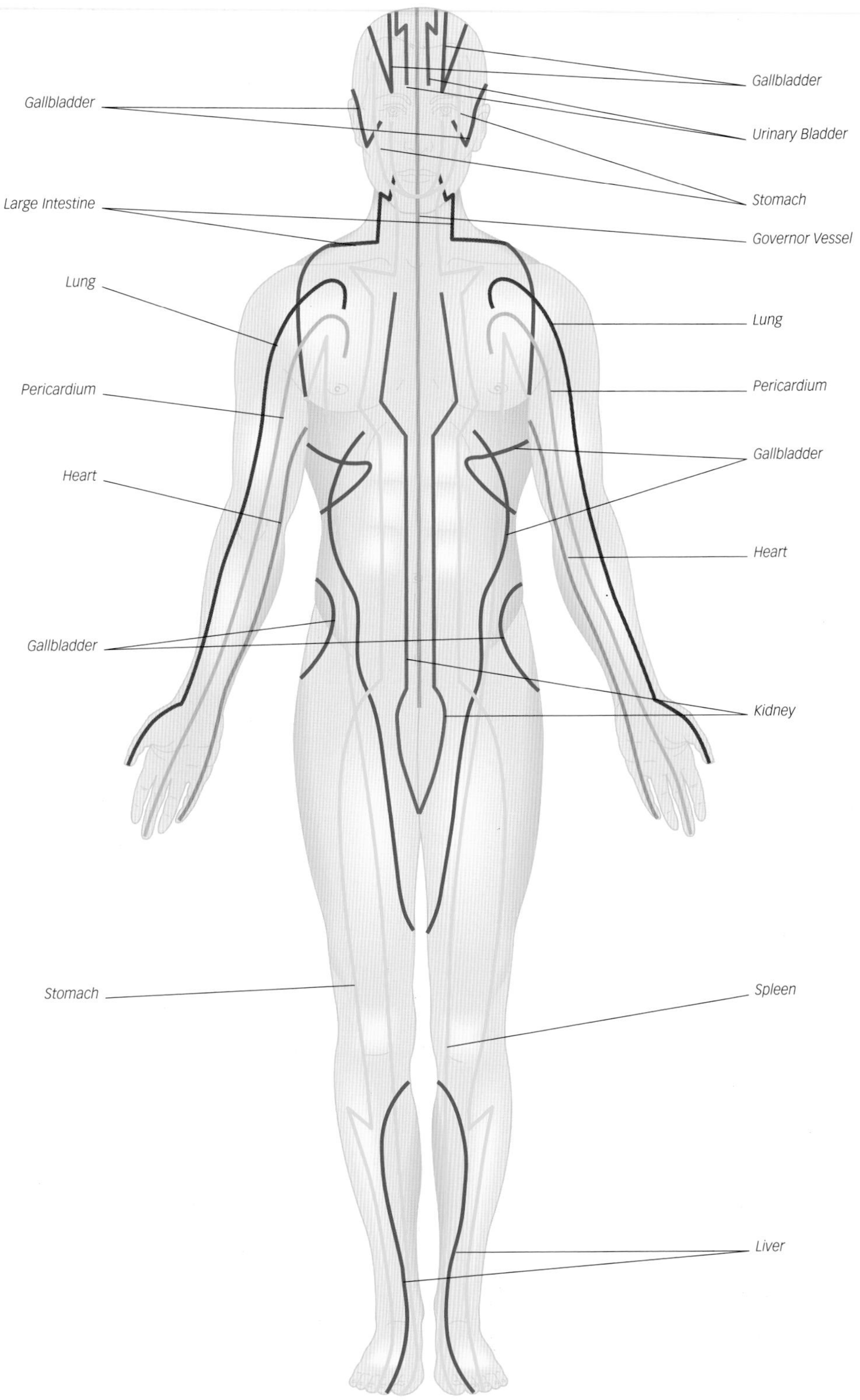

Gallbladder

Gallbladder

Urinary Bladder

Stomach

Large Intestine

Governor Vessel

Lung

Lung

Pericardium

Pericardium

Heart

Gallbladder

Gallbladder

Heart

Gallbladder

Kidney

Stomach

Spleen

Liver

THE MERIDIANS - BACK VIEW

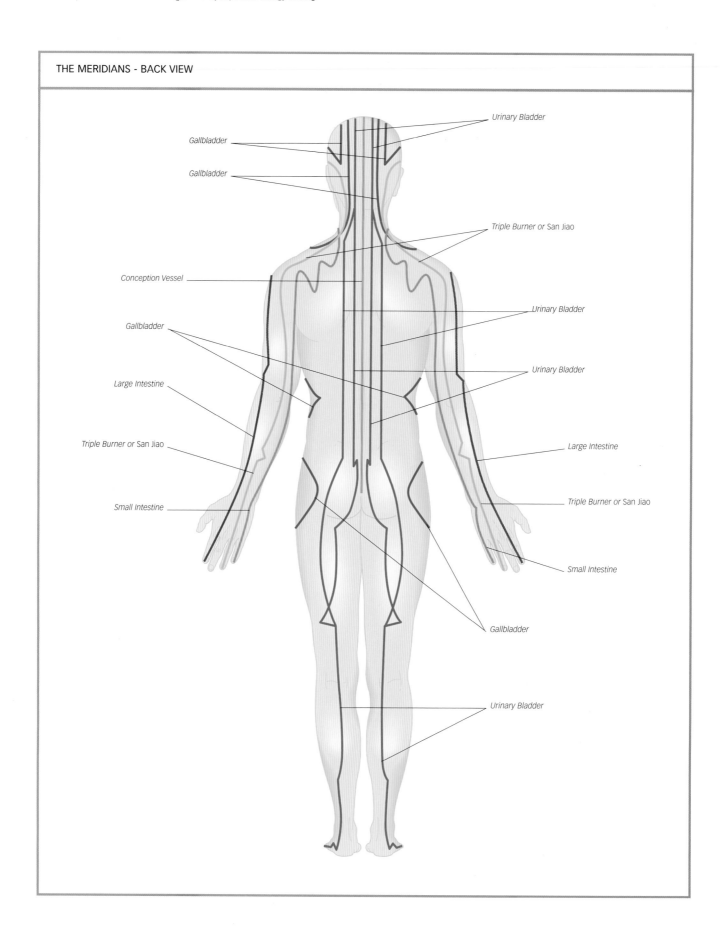

Urinary Bladder

Gallbladder

Gallbladder

Triple Burner or San Jiao

Conception Vessel

Urinary Bladder

Gallbladder

Urinary Bladder

Large Intestine

Large Intestine

Triple Burner or San Jiao

Triple Burner or San Jiao

Small Intestine

Small Intestine

Gallbladder

Urinary Bladder

tendons (muscle and tendon problems are related to the liver) and opens into the eyes. Its corresponding yang meridian is the gallbladder.

The spleen: This meridian provides energy for digestion and controls the transportation and transformation of nutrients. Its energy helps to hold the blood within the blood vessels (excessive bruising or nosebleeds are related to the spleen). It opens into the mouth. Its corresponding yang meridian is the stomach.

The kidneys: This meridian controls the body fluids, separating the pure from the impure. It controls the brain and nervous system and opens into the ears. Its corresponding yang meridian is the urinary bladder.

The lungs: This meridian controls the whole respiratory process as well as the skin and hair (eczema and other skin problems are related to the lungs). The meridian opens into the nose and its corresponding yang meridian is the large intestine.

The pericardium: This meridian protects the heart and is often used to help heart-related problems such as angina, chest complaints, and canker sores on the tongue. Its corresponding yang organ has no English anatomical equivalent but is called San Jiao or the triple burner.

The energy flowing through each meridian ebbs and flows over a 24-hour period. Each meridian has a time when its energy is at its highest flow and another when it is at its lowest ebb. Ideally, if an organ is weak it should be treated at the time when its corresponding meridian is at its highest flow. Conversely, if an organ is overworking, treating at a time when its corresponding meridian is at its lowest ebb can calm its energy the best.

MERIDIAN EBBS AND FLOWS

Meridian	Highest Flow	Lowest Ebb
Lung	3–5am	3–5pm
Large intestine	5–7am	5–7pm
Stomach	7–9am	7–9pm
Spleen	9–11am	9–11pm
Heart	11am–1pm	11pm–1am
Small intestine	1–3pm	1–3am
Urinary bladder	3–5pm	3–5am
Kidney	7–9pm	7–9am
Pericardium	9–11pm	9–11am
San Jiao	11pm–1am	11am–1pm
Gall-bladder	1–3am	1–3pm
Liver	3–5am	3–5pm

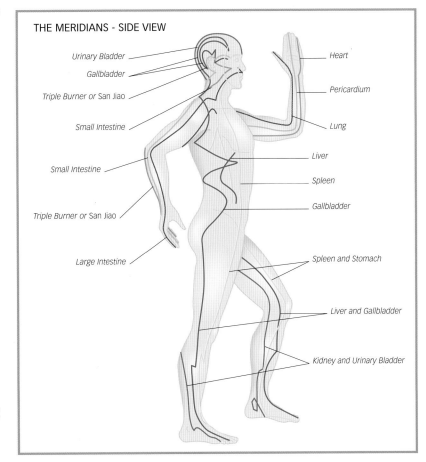

THE MERIDIANS - SIDE VIEW

Urinary Bladder
Gallbladder
Triple Burner or San Jiao
Small Intestine
Small Intestine
Triple Burner or San Jiao
Large Intestine

Heart
Pericardium
Lung
Liver
Spleen
Gallbladder
Spleen and Stomach
Liver and Gallbladder
Kidney and Urinary Bladder

3 precious energy

You are not born with an unlimited supply of energy. Your life force is finite and the manner in which you run your life has a direct effect on its state. Your life force is the precious energy without which you cannot live. When you run out of life force, you die. There are fortunately many things you can do to save and accumulate this precious energy. Unfortunately, because of the laws of yin and yang, there are also an equal and opposite amount of things you can do to deplete it.

Modern living puts great strain on the body and has a tendency to deplete life force. To maintain health, we must learn the best way to handle these strains and find ways to accumulate more energy. Learning about energy provides us with a guide to running our lives for maximum health and fulfillment.

Stress

Negative stress has an extremely detrimental effect on our energy. There is such a thing as positive stress – it is the type of stress that we feel when we set ourselves goals and targets which we then achieve. This is known as "eu-stress" and it is actually good for us since it increases our inner strength and determination. Negative stress is called "dis-stress" and does us nothing but harm.

Stress usually falls into one of four areas:
1 Work: Too much or too little work is not good for one's health. We all need to work in some way or another to maintain healthy bodies but too much or too little depletes energy. If your work causes you stress, you need to look at what it will take to make your job better. Learning time management skills can often reduce work pressure. If you do not like your job then the obvious thing to do is to find a new job, but that is often easier said

than done. Learn to change your attitude to your job since stress is actually caused by how we react to our work, not by the work itself.
2 Home: This should be a place of rest and relaxation for all the family, including the homemaker. Relaxation is an essential process that allows our bodies to heal and rejuvenate. Relaxation does not just mean sitting in front of the television, it means giving both mind and body time to rest and rebalance.
3 Self-expression: Lack of freedom or an inability to express oneself and one's emotions is an area of stress that we often ignore. It is not good to bottle things up. We all need some form of self-expression if we are to feel fulfilled. If your freedom is restricted to the detriment of your health, it is vital you find an alternative way to express yourself – perhaps through art or writing.
4 Social interaction: We all need to meet and converse with other human beings. It is one of the greatest ways of learning through the exchange of knowledge and experience. A solitary existence is usually an unhappy one. Conversely, too much socializing can be detrimental if it leads to stress in one of the other three areas.

RIGHT Try to find a time and a place to relax properly. Avoid the distractions at home by sitting in a park.

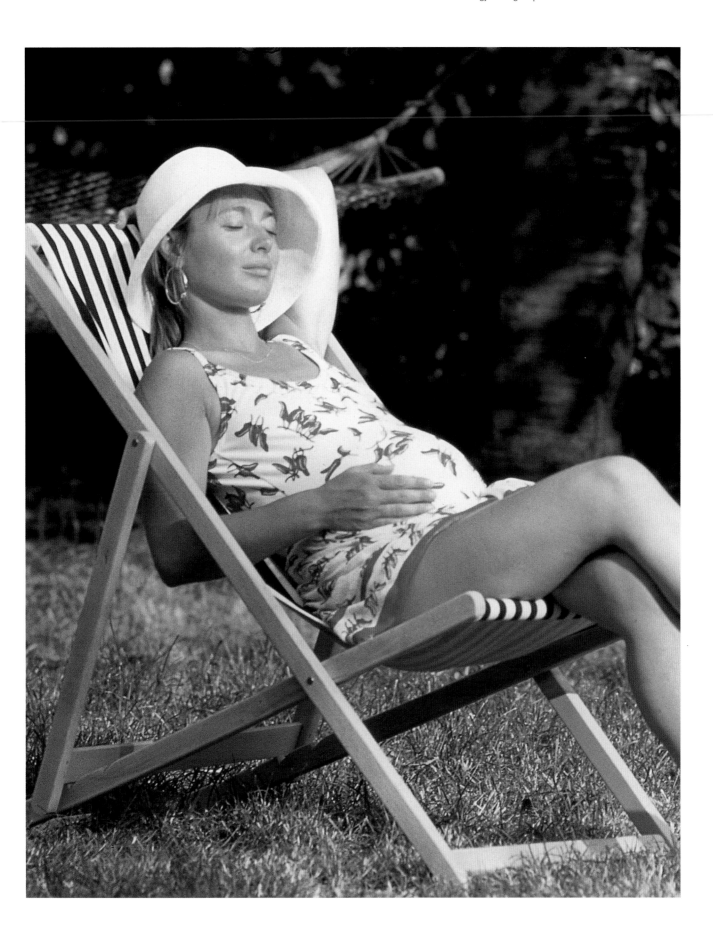

Modern living

Modern living provides our bodies with endless stresses and strains. The way we choose to run our lives contributes greatly to our ill health. It is only by looking at ways to change and improve our living that we can hope to find true health and happiness. There is a tendency in the West to resist change. We even have a saying, "Better the devil you know, than the devil you don't," which basically means "I would rather stick with my unpleasant life because if I try to change it, it might get even worse." This is a self-limiting philosophy and we in the West are experts at producing them.

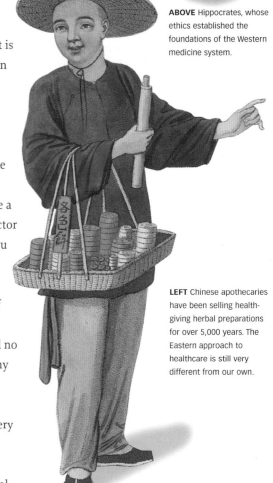

ABOVE Hippocrates, whose ethics established the foundations of the Western medicine system.

Another self-limiting philosophy is, "The illness you have is incurable." Believing in this statement stops people searching for the health and happiness that is their birthright. There is no such thing as an incurable disease unless you choose to believe what some doctors tell you. Just because no known cure can be found for a particular disease in the West does not mean that a cure cannot be found anywhere in the world.

In certain parts of China, there used to be a healthcare system where you paid your doctor all the time you were well. The moment you became ill, you stopped paying and did not start paying again until you were fully restored to health. How the effectiveness of Western medicine would change if that philosophy was adopted here. Drugs would no longer be the primary therapy because many drugs have side effects that lead to more ill health. Doctors would have to search for solutions rather than using drugs and surgery in an attempt to eradicate symptoms.

Until relatively recent times, Western doctors took the Hippocratic oath, an ethical

LEFT Chinese apothecaries have been selling health-giving herbal preparations for over 5,000 years. The Eastern approach to healthcare is still very different from our own.

charter of medical conduct created by the great Greek physician, Hippocrates. Part of the oath states: "I will follow that system of regimen which, according to my ability and judgement, I consider for the benefit of my patients, and abstain from whatever is deleterious and mischievous. I will give no deadly medicine to anyone if asked, nor suggest any such counsel." Some modern medical drugs are so toxic that it would be impossible for any doctor who prescribed them to be faithful to this oath. There are many avenues of medicine to be explored and if more doctors decide to explore them, Western medicine will one day again be able to embody the spirit of this oath once more.

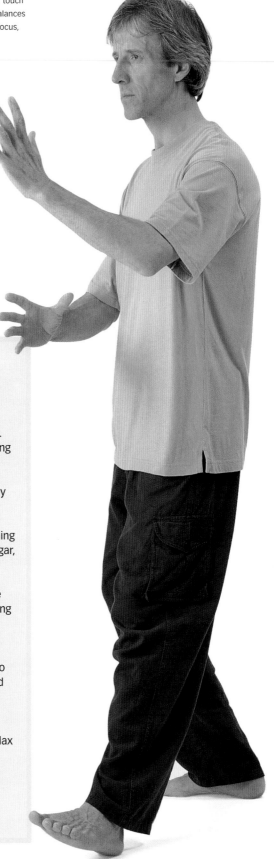

RIGHT Regular tai chi puts you in touch with the needs of your body. It balances the emotions, heightens mental focus, and releases creativity.

THE DIFFERENCE IN EASTERN AND WESTERN LIFESTYLES

Sleep is a great healer because it allows the body's energies time to rebuild and balance. After a good night's sleep, you wake up with an energy surplus that helps to get you up and sustains you through the day. In the East, when people wake up in this state, they then spend their day building more energy. In the West, when people wake up in this state, they spend their day squandering it.

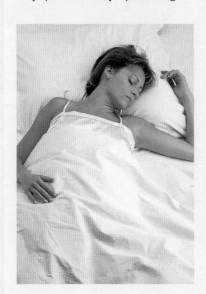

East – Wake up and begin the day with an energy-building exercise (i.e. tai chi) followed by a simple energy-building food and drink (i.e. simply cooked grain, energy-building herbal tea).

West – Wake up and begin the day with no exercise or an energy depleting exercise (i.e. jogging) followed by complex energy-draining food and drink (i.e. cereal with sugar, meat, coffee etc.).

East – Work hard, eat simply, take breaks to allow time for rebalancing mind and body.

West – Work hard, eat complex foods, take breaks to allow time to eat and drink energy-draining food and drink (sugar-filled snacks and more coffee!).

East – Come home to rest and relax with a simple, balanced meal.

West – Come home to watch TV and eat energy-draining foods.

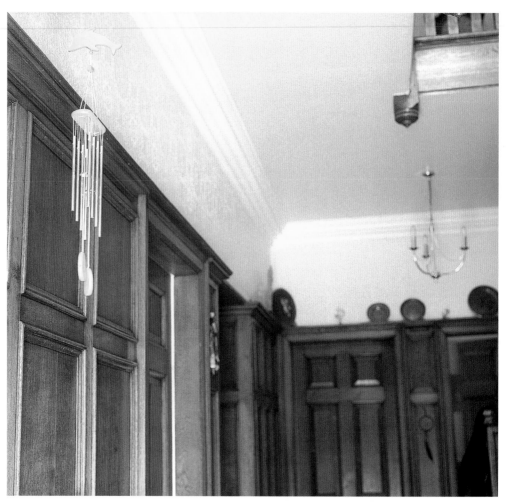

RIGHT A hallway is filled with moving energies as the inhabitants of a house pass through without stopping. According to feng shui, metal wind chimes balance the space by slowing down fast chi.

Geopathic stress

In this modern, technologically advanced age, we are surrounded with unnatural substances and energies that can cause our bodies to become imbalanced. This kind of stress is called geopathic stress and it refers to such things as radiation and chemical toxins. Our bodies rely on biochemical processes to function and many of these processes involve chemicals within the body acting like magnets to attract other chemicals. When a human exposes him- or herself to strong electrical fields, the natural biochemical processes become confused and interrupted.

The magnetic influence of radiation on our foods and bodies acts like a slow energy drain. Many people accept that living underneath an electricity pylon is not good for your health, but do not realize that they spend much of their time sitting inside other strong electromagnetic fields and eating irradiated food. If you sleep with an electric blanket plugged in, even if it is switched off, you will be sleeping in an electromagnetic field that will drain energy from you while you sleep. Microwaving, "the fast solution for busy people" is an unnatural way of cooking that fills the food with radiation and renders many of the nutrients within that food indigestible. Computers, televisions, and cell phones all give off low levels of radiation that can, over time, be detrimental to your health. This does not mean that you have to abandon electricity, just that you may need to modify your lifestyle so that you are less exposed to such things.

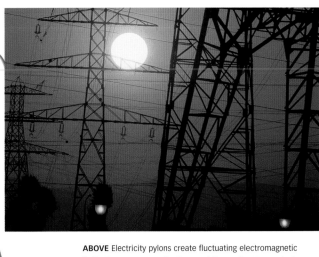

ABOVE Electricity pylons create fluctuating electromagnetic fields that can cause migraines and depression. Use an ionizer to counteract their effects inside your home.

stress, but often a few simple things can help to counteract it. Wind chimes help to keep energy moving in your home and spider plants are particularly good at improving overall energy levels because they release rich amounts of oxygen. Amethyst can help to counteract radiation, and lots of plants improve oxygen levels. If you feel your home is draining your energy, perhaps you might like to contact a professional dowser or feng shui practitioner to locate the root causes of your problem. A dowser will use a pendulum to check the flow of energy within a house. A feng shui practitioner uses the ancient Chinese five-element theory to check the energetic balance within the house.

LEFT Spider plants absorb gases from synthetic paints and carpets more effectively than mechanical filters, creating a healthier environment.

- If you have wires around and under your bed, make sure you unplug them before you go to sleep.
- If you work at a computer, take regular breaks (at least 10 minutes every hour).
- If you use a cell phone, keep calls as short as possible, change listening ears at regular intervals, and never use it within the metal framework of a car.
- If you have a microwave, stop using it!

Many modern houses are full of geopathic

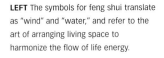

LEFT The symbols for feng shui translate as "wind" and "water," and refer to the art of arranging living space to harmonize the flow of life energy.

Healthy and unhealthy energy

Throughout our lives we come into contact with a multitude of different energies. Some energies are good for us and help us on our path toward health and happiness, other energies cause imbalance and slow us down on our path. These energies are not necessarily "bad" because within every negative is an equal and opposite amount of positive which can be found if you look for it.

Life is full of opportunities to learn. When a child is told by its parent not to go near the flame it often ignores the advice and suffers a small, but very traumatic, burn. Through that negative experience the child learns a healthy respect for fire that will undoubtedly save its life several times over. This is the positive lesson to be found within the negative experience.

Life is full of such experiences. If someone treats you badly, you can become bitter and angry, which is not a healthy state to be in, or you can try to learn from the experience. If you do learn from it, you can then go to the person who was horrible to you and say, "Thank you for the way you treated me. Because of your actions, I have had to look within myself and have learned many lessons from them. You have helped me to become a better and wiser person and I can only be grateful." This is how to turn negative to positive.

Everything you experience in life, including illness, is an opportunity to become better and wiser. If you embrace all of life, "good" and "bad," as a learning experience, life becomes an adventure of insights and realizations. Illness is just another series of lessons waiting to be learned. Seek those lessons diligently, strong in the knowledge that with each passing day and with each new experience you are becoming a wiser, better, and stronger person.

BELOW Lack of sleep often contributes to feelings of anxiety and depression, so a good night's sleep is essential for both physical and mental well-being.

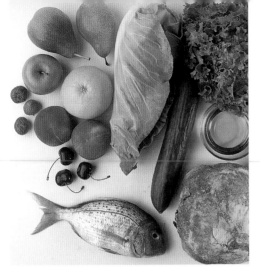

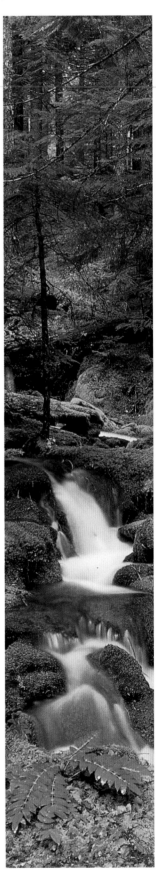

LEFT A nutritious diet full of fresh additive-free foods, especially organic fruit and vegetables, can help you cope with negative emotions such as depression, fear, and anxiety. Adzuki beans (opposite page) are particularly beneficial for the kidneys, the organs linked to the emotion fear.

RIGHT To alleviate feelings of depression, seek environments that are uplifting or calming – take a walk by a beautiful woodland waterfall. Try to spend more time doing things that make you feel good.

Healing energy-draining emotions

Emotions such as fear, worry, depression, and anger are manifestations of imbalance within the body. These simple self-help aids can help overcome these emotions. They are not quick-fix solutions, but signposts to guide you toward long-term solutions.

Fear: This emotion is strongly linked to the kidneys. The more grounded you are, the less you will be troubled by fear. Eat natural foods and lots of root vegetables. Adzuki beans are very good for the kidneys and so help to control fear. Develop more power within yourself by gently stretching yourself (i.e. setting yourself tasks of increasing challenge).

Depression: This emotion is linked to the heart. Seek environments that are uplifting, share love, and be around nature. Eat healthily and get plenty of sleep. Comfort eating never provides a long-term solution, that solution can only be found within you.

Worry and anxiety: This emotion is linked to the lungs and the thyroid gland. Worry stems from a sense of not having the resources to cope with certain situations (often the "resource" is money). Whatever resource it is you are lacking, the only way you can find it is by continuing to search and learn from all experiences. Live in the present and try to learn from life's experiences.

Anger: This emotion is linked to the liver. Anger is caused by a lack of healthy energy expression. We are expressive beings who need to express our lives in a fulfilling way. If we fail to do this, frustration builds within and manifests as anger without.

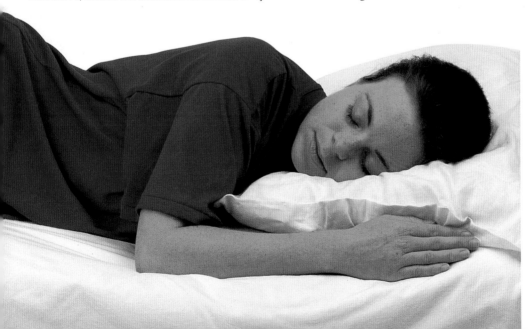

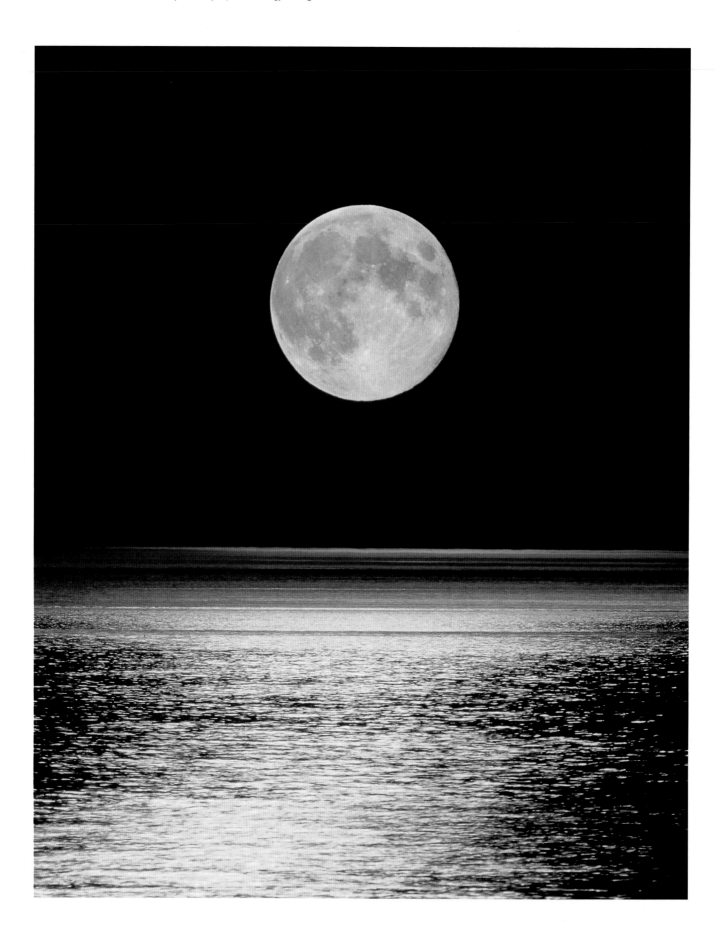

How natural phenomena affect our health

The full moon: The moon not only affects the tides but all fluids on the earth, including all body fluids. The full moon seems to have a particularly strong effect on humans. The word "lunacy" comes from the word "lunar" and was often called "moon-madness." The full moon tends to make children more hyperactive and admissions to mental hospitals tend to be highest around the full moon.

Barometric pressure: When barometric pressure falls, body fluids become thicker and this can aggravate asthma, arthritis, depression, diabetes, epilepsy, migraines and headaches, pain, and ulcers.

Wind temperatures and directions: The following ailments are aggravated by different types of winds. Warm southerly winds aggravate allergies, lung problems (i.e. asthma, bronchitis), depression, circulatory problems

LEFT The metal tubes of wind chimes slow energy flow. Energy passing between the chimes is refined by their sound.

(i.e. angina) and insomnia. Warm westerly winds aggravate anaemia, colitis, epilepsy, migraines, liver ailments, and depression. Cold northerly winds aggravate diabetes, arthritis, rheumatism, and kidney ailments. Cold westerly winds aggravate cramps, arthritis, muscle ailments, and rheumatism.

Thunderstorms: These create massive amounts of electricity in the air, filling it with an excess of positively charged ions. This excess can cause depression, dulling of mental abilities, and a general feeling of being "under the weather." Once the storm has passed there is an equal and opposite excess of negatively charged ions. The negative charge has the effect of improving mental function and lifting the spirits.

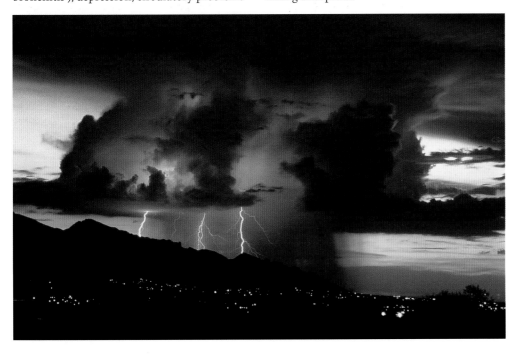

LEFT Storms are natural ionizers: lightning produces negative ions, replacing those destroyed by central heating, synthetic fibers, and electrical appliances. Ionizing effects occur after the storm has passed.

FAR LEFT Some astrologers can predict potential illnesses from the position of the planets at the moment of birth.

Shen, chi, and jing

To be happy, healthy, and fulfilled you need to have "good" shen, chi, and jing. Shen is a sense of love and upliftedness; chi is energy; and jing is essence. If everyone sought to have good shen, chi, and jing there would be little or no ill health in the world. Neither would there be wars or crime. Mankind would find its true destiny and live in a state of happiness, health, and fulfillment. This would truly create heaven on earth.

Shen

A life devoid of love is a life devoid of happiness. You should always seek to do everything with love. You reap what you sow; so if you give out love, you will naturally attract love back to yourself. This "love" is a love that is unconditional and universal. It is not our place to judge other people, only to love them. Do all things from a perspective of genuine care for all human life.

A high quality practitioner of medicine, regardless of their specific discipline, should always work from a perspective of love. This includes all complementary health practitioners, doctors, surgeons, nurses, counselors, and everyone else involved in health and healthcare. In your search for health, happiness, and fulfillment, anyone you meet who lacks shen will not be good for you. Love is the most fundamental of all human emotions and is therefore a fundamental requirement for everyone to have in their lives if they are to be happy.

Chi

To be healthy, one needs good chi. Human beings are naturally expressive and a good free flow of energy is essential for health. Blockages in our energy pathways lead to ill health. You can tell if someone has good chi. They have an "energy" about them that is attractive and pleasant to experience. They are the sort of people you like to be around because they make you feel good. People who drain your energy, who leave you feeling tired or depressed do not have good chi.

All healthcare practitioners should have good chi. Sadly, many doctors, nurses, and complementary practitioners are so

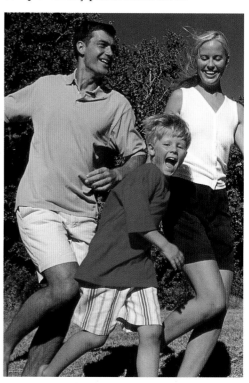

RIGHT Good energy flow is essential for health, and exercise helps to balance the flow. When we good, we boost the energy of those around us.

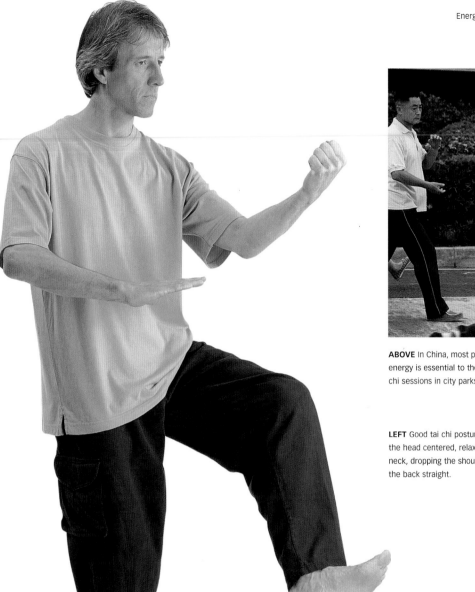

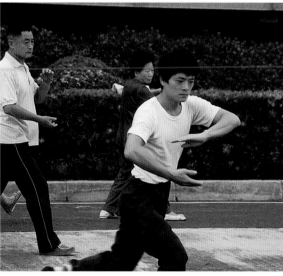

ABOVE In China, most people understand that maintaining a good flow of life energy is essential to their health and well-being. Anyone can join in group tai chi sessions in city parks.

LEFT Good tai chi posture includes keeping the head centered, relaxing the face and neck, dropping the shoulders, and keeping the back straight.

overworked and drained by their patients that they do not always have good chi. Hopefully, as the Western understanding of energy and energy healing increases, there will come a time when everyone is taught how to maintain a good level of chi.

Jing

Jing is the life force within each and every one of us. Without it we cease to exist and yet in the West we seem to do many things that deplete our Jing. Bad diet and poor quality of life deplete jing and people in the West are eating more and more unhealthily and creating more negative emotions and stresses in their lives. No wonder illness is reaching such high levels. To be truly fulfilled, you should be increasing your jing.

It is very hard for a normal individual to perceive the state of another's jing. All health practitioners should be actively building jing and teaching their patients how to build jing. In China it is fundamental to all traditional healthcare. Anyone who is ill is taught how to build their jing through the practice of tai chi or chi kung. Some of these exercises are very simple to learn and can be practiced by anyone (see Chi kung pages 90–93).

Using energy healing to restore balance

No matter what illness you may suffer from, energy-healing techniques can help by restoring balance and harmony in your life. As you read through Part 2 of this book, some therapies will appeal to you more than others. This is your intuition telling you which therapies can potentially help you on your search for true health, happiness, and fulfillment. This does not mean that therapies that do not appeal to you at this time should be totally rejected. On the contrary, it just means that those therapies are not right for you at this time – they may well be right for you in the future.

If there are many therapies that appeal to you, the best way to narrow down the options is to learn more about each of the therapies. Some therapies work well together, while others can work antagonistically, so trying them all is not necessarily the wisest course of action. Consult some of the many books about the different aspects of energy healing and find out about the many things you can do to help balance your own energy.

Finding a therapist

All energy healers should be willing to talk to you about their work and should do so with enthusiasm. If that spark of enthusiasm is not there, the therapist will probably have poor shen, chi, and jing and will not be good for your energy. A therapist should always be willing to talk openly and honestly about their experience and their success rate. Although it is a bonus if a therapist has had firsthand experience of treating a specific ailment, it is not essential. What is more important is their approach and attitude. If they are bright, enthusiastic, and work from a perspective of unconditional love (good shen), if they are vibrant with energy (good chi), and if they

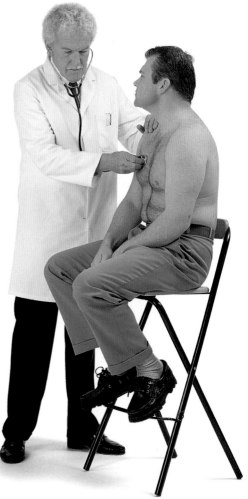

ABOVE In Western medicine, an examination will usually concentrate on physical symptoms. A good doctor will take the time to talk to his or her patients, because their own intuition will often indicate the root of a physical problem.

appear fulfilled in their lives (good jing), then they cannot help but do you good regardless of their experience of a specific problem.

One of the best ways to find a good quality therapist is by word of mouth. A personal recommendation is always preferable to random choice. If you can find someone who has received good treatment from a practitioner in the field you are seeking, that is often the best way to proceed. Just because a therapist belongs to a registry does not necessarily mean that they are guaranteed to be a high quality practitioner. Equally, not being on a register does not indicate a low quality practitioner.

Focusing your thoughts on finding a good quality therapist will help you to attract one into your life. This, combined with using your intuition, researching and questioning, will help you on your path to finding the therapist who is best for you. As a rule of thumb, always check out their shen, chi, and jing before you book yourself in. It is often worth seeing a Western doctor before consulting an alternative therapist if only to obtain an accurate diagnosis and to rule out serious, undiscovered illness or at least to be aware of it.

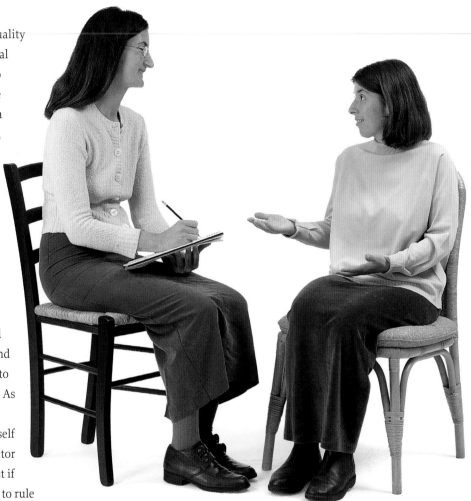

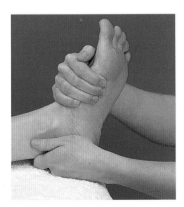

ABOVE Reflexology maps out the major systems of the body on the soles of the feet and improves energy flow in the whole body.

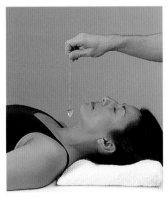

ABOVE Dowsing locates negative energy. A pendulum is held over the body and will indicate the patient's imbalances by the direction and quality of its swing.

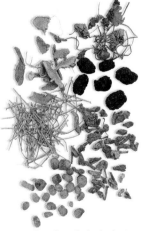

ABOVE Plants form the basis of many modern drugs, and are used in their pure form in Chinese and Ayurvedic medicine and Western herbalism.

ABOVE An alternative therapist will ask questions to build up a mental and physical picture of you. Holistic therapy treats the whole person, not just a set of symptoms.

Destiny

The path to health, happiness, and fulfillment is one and the same with the path of destiny. Destiny is a strange concept for many Westerners but it can best be explained as the most efficient path of learning for you. Our life purpose is to learn from all our experiences and thus become better and wiser individuals. If we are willing to learn from all our experiences, the fundamental thing we learn is how to attract more positive things into our lives and fewer negative ones.

As you progress through life, some things that you do give you a sense of fulfillment; these are part of your unfolding path toward health, and happiness. Other things leave you cold or dissatisfied. These things are to be avoided in the future wherever possible. In this way, you will gradually tailor your life toward peace, harmony, and balance.

Every human being has a right to do what they really want to do. Every human being has the right to live the life of their dreams. This means that if you set forth a dream in your mind of how you want your life to be, then you have the power within you to make that dream reality. If you keep your intent focused on your dream, everything you encounter, positive or negative, will be a stepping stone closer to the realization of that dream. Every obstacle will be a lesson waiting to be learned. Part of everybody's dream can be to be happy, healthy, and fulfilled. This does not mean that overnight you will be healed of all your ills. What it means is that if you make total health a part of your dream, as you search for that dream, you will encounter lessons that will help you to come ever closer to the realization of that dream. This is the path of destiny that we can all choose to tread.

Scenario 1

Imagine you meet a psychic who is never wrong. The psychic tells you about many aspects of your life that only you know about and is so accurate that you believe everything that they tell you. This is not foolishness in this situation because the psychic is not only highly gifted, but also totally honorable. Then one day the psychic tells you that they have received a message for you saying that you have only six months left to live. Nothing else in your life changes and it doesn't matter what you do, in six months time you will disincarnate. What would you do?

Scenario 2

A long-lost relative dies and leaves you a fortune. What would you do? If you can honestly answer these two questions with, "I would change nothing" then you are probably already living the life of your dreams. If not, look at the things you would do in these two situations. Chances are they are part of your dream and if so, set them firmly in your mind, keep searching, and you will find a way to make them reality.

Forming a dream

Many people have trouble working out what they would really like to do with their lives. There are endless possibilities but people and situations often distract us from connecting to our dream. The two main things that seem to stop Westerners from doing what they really want are time and money, which lead us to losing sight of our destiny. The two scenarios to the left remove these factors and help you to focus on what you would really like to do.

RIGHT Imagine that a deep river separates you from the life you want. Create stepping stones by taking one small action every day toward your dreams.

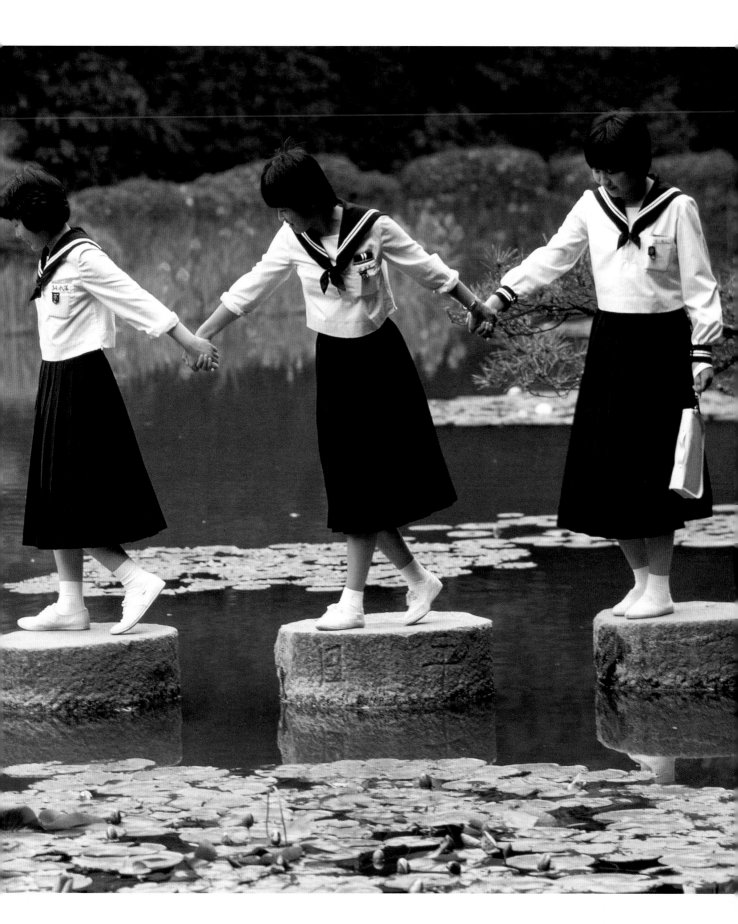

Guidelines for treating illness

All illness is the body's way of trying to tell you that you are not doing something as well or as healthily as you could. Once you have learned the lessons your body is trying to teach you, you have no reason to manifest the illness any more. Some illnesses teach simple truths and others teach lessons on many different levels. Generally, the more serious the illness, the more you can potentially learn from it.

Anyone who is ill in any way should always look at his or her diet. Good nutrition is fundamental to health and well-being. Everyone can also benefit from learning some form of energy-building exercise since this will not only stop energy blockages but also help to build jing (life force). After that, it is best to try therapies individually because you can then judge each one on its own merits. Often one has to explore several therapies to bring about total healing but each one contributes in its own way and has its own lessons to teach.

The most important thing is never to stop searching for solutions to your problems. Never accept that you cannot have the life of your dreams. If you set your sights on

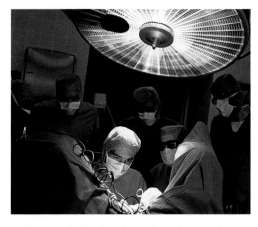

ABOVE Surgery is often the last resort for Western medicine, but holistic medicine has much to offer.

50 percent health, the best you will ever achieve is 50 percent health. You will never be able to achieve 60, 70, 80, or 90 percent. If you set your sights on 100 per cent health, happiness, and fulfillment, you are setting no limits on what you can achieve and you will be more likely to find the life of your dreams.

The limits of Western medicine

In general, Western medicine has two main therapies: medicinal drugs and surgery. This means that if the illness you

LEFT Make sure your diet consists of fresh, natural foods packed with essential vitamins and minerals. A constant diet of refined foods, stimulants, and additives can lead to illness in the long term.

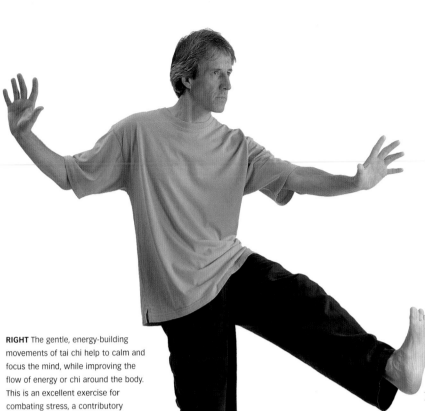

RIGHT The gentle, energy-building movements of tai chi help to calm and focus the mind, while improving the flow of energy or chi around the body. This is an excellent exercise for combating stress, a contributory factor in some serious diseases, including cancer.

have does not respond to either therapy, often it is labeled as "incurable." This is a self-limiting philosophy and if you choose to believe it you are choosing to abandon your dreams. There are endless recorded cases of people being healed from supposedly incurable diseases, including arthritis, irritable bowel syndrome, epilepsy, ME, and cancer to name but a few. In most cases the healing has come as a result of a journey that encompasses many different and diverse therapies. The one thing that all these individuals have in common is that they never stopped searching for answers.

This does not mean that you should immediately abandon Western medicine. What it does mean is that if Western medicine does not provide all of the answers that you are seeking, do not be afraid to look elsewhere. Better still, try to persuade your family doctor to help you on your journey of discovery and to give you their wisdom and counsel. The

BELOW Western medicine does not always have the answers – many alternative therapies are available.

more doctors begin to search with their patients for answers outside drugs and surgery, the healthier the West will become. Likewise, if you have found benefit from an alternative therapy then tell your physician about it. In this way we will be a step closer to a fully integrated medical system where the patient's health is placed over and above all other considerations (including money, time, and other resources).

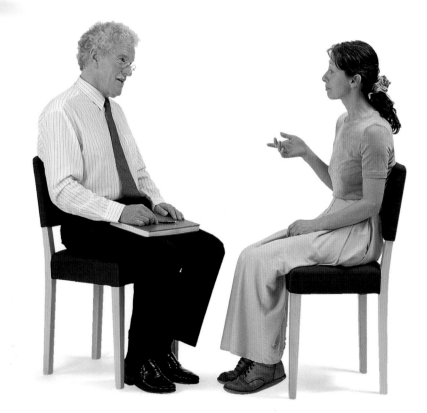

A holistic approach to cancer

Cancer is one of the most prevalent and feared of all Western diseases. Much of this fear has been created by our own imbalance and can be banished by a simple change in attitude. Cancer is no different from any other disease in the sense that it is just another way of your body trying to teach you. Once you understand this, you can get on with the job of learning and thus curing your cancer.

The Chinese definition of cancer is "stagnant chi and blood," which is very apt because everyone who has cancer is "stuck" in one or more areas of their lives. This means part of the curing of cancer is linked to the "un-sticking" of those areas and the best way to do this is to initiate change in your life. Not change for change's sake, but change from unhealthy to healthy practices.

Factors that can lead to cancer

Nutrition: The most common factor is faulty nutrition and/or vitamin and mineral deficiency. This is not resolved by simply popping lots of vitamin and mineral supplements.

Radiation: It is widely accepted that radiation is a cause of cancer. What is not widely accepted, but is nonetheless true, is that accumulated radiation from electrical equipment such as cell phones, microwaves, excessive X rays, televisions, electric blankets, wires under the bed, and power lines can all be contributory factors to cancer. Even much of our food is now irradiated to make it stay "fresh" longer!

Free radicals: There are growing concerns about hydrogenation of food, chlorination of water, many food packaging materials such as plastic wrappings, and other supposedly "safe" practices that fill our bodies with tiny chemical magnets (called "free radicals"). These latch on to many of the vitamins and minerals in our food, rendering them inert and indigestible.

Toxins in the food chain: Much of our food is full of toxins (chemical additives, genetically modified organisms, pesticide residues, heavy metals etc.) that act as a slow poison to our systems.

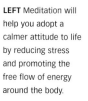

LEFT Meditation will help you adopt a calmer attitude to life by reducing stress and promoting the free flow of energy around the body.

Emotional and spiritual blockages:
Unresolved emotional baggage (i. e. guilt, anger, resentment etc.) and ignored spiritual needs can both contribute to cancer.

Lack of time: Being too busy to look after all your personal needs.

Treating cancer

Use cancer as a learning experience. Approach it with curiosity rather than fear. Treat the disease with respect, not hatred, for however unwelcome it may be, it is a part of your life. Eat nutritious foods and become an expert on health and healthy living. Take up one or more energy-building exercises and learn to use your mind to help heal your body. Learn to release all negative thoughts and find a purpose in your life that resonates deep within your being. Search for solutions rather than focusing on problems. Learn to still yourself. Seek that which will help to make you happy, healthy, and fulfilled. Learn to trust your intuition. Have courage and learn to give and receive healing. Always make up your own mind.

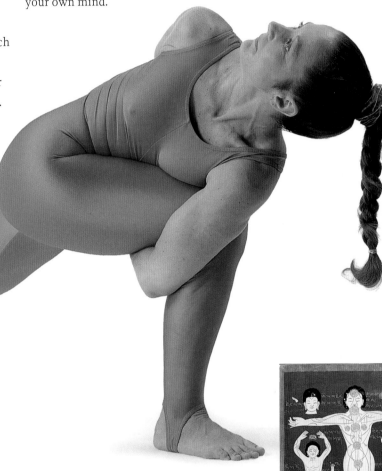

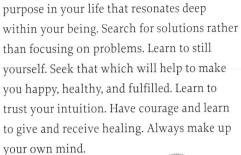

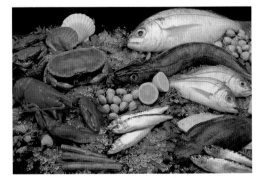

ABOVE Energy-building exercises, such as yoga, are wonderful for releasing energy blockages caused by stress. In the long term these blockages may manifest themselves as cancer.

ABOVE Fish provide a rich source of vitamins A, D, and B$_6$. Research has shown that a nutritionally poor diet lacking in essential vitamins and minerals can lead to ill health.

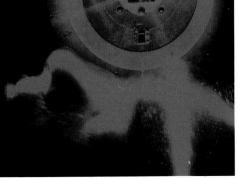

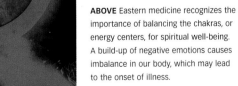

ABOVE Eastern medicine recognizes the importance of balancing the chakras, or energy centers, for spiritual well-being. A build-up of negative emotions causes imbalance in our body, which may lead to the onset of illness.

LEFT A patient with a brain tumor undergoing radiation treatment – a conventional method for treating cancer.

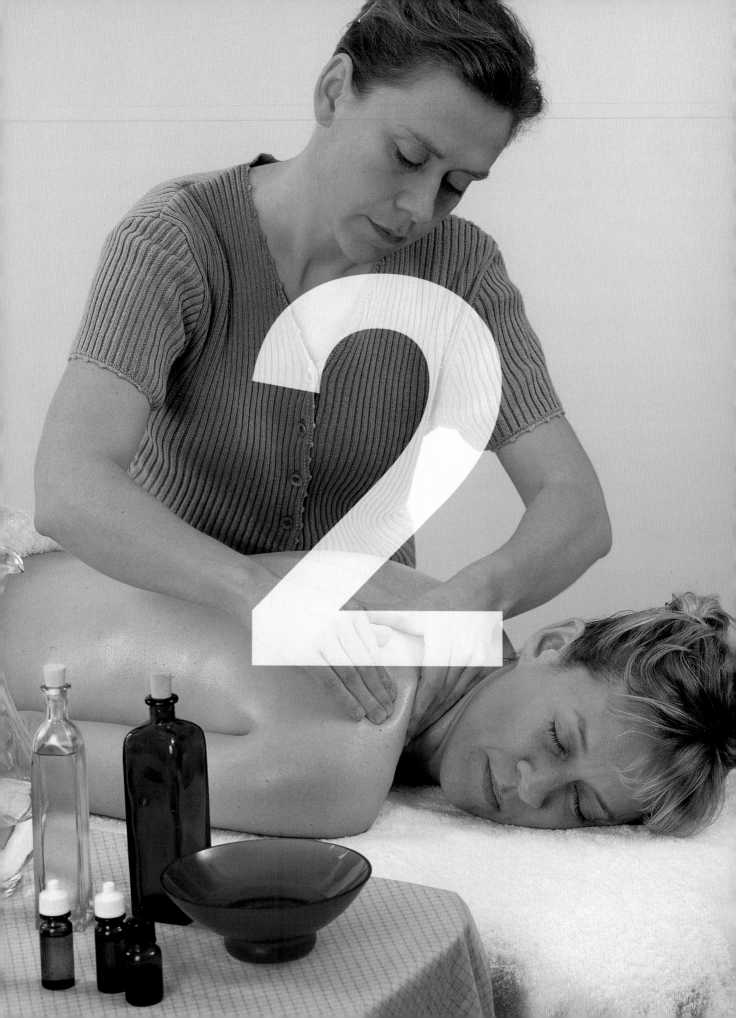

healing energies

This part of the book provides an overview of the main therapies in the field of energy healing. The emphasis throughout is on how to receive high quality healing and teaching. Some sections offer advice on finding a high quality therapist, though this is a difficult thing to give advice on, because there are so many aspects that need to be addressed when searching for a therapist or teacher. However, there are general points that apply to all therapists and some that are specific to individual therapies. Where specific qualities are called for, they are clearly described.

The most important thing to remember is that all therapists should be open and honest. They should radiate love and warmth and have a genuine interest in you and your health. They should be willing to answer any question that you may ask and should never need to defend their therapy.

The field of energy healing is diverse and fascinating. If explored with an open mind, it can show you not only how to be happy, healthy, and fulfilled, but it can also show you great wisdom, which can have a positive effect on everyone you meet. You have the power to change lives, but that change can only become reality if you first change yourself. All the answers to your health problems lie within you. None of these therapies will magically restore you to health. They all require you to be an active participant in your search for health, happiness, and fulfillment. If you are looking for someone else to do all the work, you will never find health.

These therapies can help you to bring about positive change within yourself if you are willing to embrace that change, but if you hold on to negative thoughts and behavioral patterns, they will only give you, at best, short-term symptomatic relief. It is your birthright to find health and balance, but you must actively claim that birthright for it to become reality.

Food and water

The two most fundamental things that sustain us are food and water. Without either we die. Food provides us with most of the energy we need to pursue our lives. You are what you eat. In the West we have lost our common sense when it comes to our nutrition. Our society is run on greed and this has directly affected our nutrition and health. We are totally orally fixated in the West and we look for food to make us feel better emotionally, rather than nourished and balanced. Modern technology has enabled us to produce cheap foods which have little or no nutritional value, yet taste absolutely delicious.

If you go into an organic food store, you will find the prices higher than in ordinary stores. This has nothing to do with the greed of the organic store owners; it has to do with the fact that it takes time and labor to produce high quality, balanced foods, and this is reflected in the price. When your local burger bar offers two burgers for the price of one, this appears to be a bargain and our sense of greed implores us to take advantage of it. This is illusion. There is virtually nothing good and healthy in

fast food and lots of bad; only unhealthy things made to taste good.

In Bejing, since the introduction of American fast foods, obesity among children has risen from zero to 10 percent and is steadily rising. This is due solely to the overconsumption of indigestible fats and toxic, synthetic chemicals in fast foods. It is being effectively treated with nothing more than a good balanced diet consisting of rice, vegetables, and white fish.

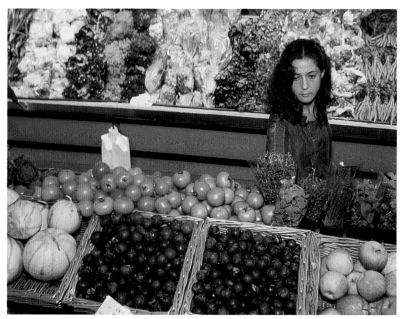

RIGHT Investigate your local health food store. Introducing organic foods that are free of chemicals and additives into your diet can help prevent disease.

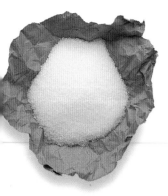

LEFT Refined white sugar has little nutritional value at all, and should be replaced with natural sweeteners, although in moderation.

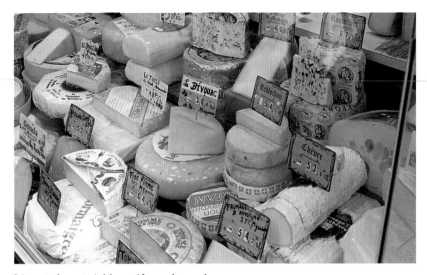

ABOVE Goat's cheese, popular in France, is less likely to trigger any allergic reactions. It contains low amounts of tyramine, a migraine-inducing chemical that is found in larger quantities in cow's cheese.

Sugar, the ultimate drug

Sugar is one of the most unbalancing and addictive refined foods to have been created by man. If you chewed a piece of sugar beet, you would find that you could do so for only a few minutes because it is too sweet. Your body naturally tells you via your taste buds when you have had enough. Once refined though, sugar loses a great deal of its sweetness and your taste buds can no longer tell you when you have had too much. Refined sugar is also one of the most addictive substances on the planet and from the moment an adult says to a child, "Stop crying and I'll give you a candy," sugar becomes a source of false comfort when we want to feel better.

Sugar is poison to the human body. Eating 5oz (150g) sugar can weaken your immune system greatly. This is because sugar is not digested in the normal way other foods are. Sugar is absorbed directly into the bloodstream via the mouth and the stomach wall. This greatly unbalances the blood sugar levels and the pancreas then has to produce massive amounts of insulin to restore the balance. While your body is using all its energy to rebalance itself, your immune system is not being fed. Sugar is the number one cause of illness in the Western world. If you want to be healthy, you should not eat refined sugar. Nature provides many natural sweeteners that are much better for you, such as rice syrup, barley malt, corn syrup, and agave syrup. Honey has long been regarded as a traditional sweetener, but many commercial honey producers add refined sugar to their hives to boost yields; so if you do use honey it is best to buy an organic one that states on the label that there is "No added sugar." But even these natural sweeteners should never be eaten to excess.

Is milk really good for you?

We are the only animals who consume milk after the weaning period. Does this really make sense? Nature made cow's milk for baby cows, not for baby humans. There is mounting evidence that one of the causes of illnesses such as asthma, eczema, and arthritis is intolerance to dairy products. Furthermore, cow's milk is not a good source of calcium for humans, not least because we combine it with sugar or coffee, which both inhibit calcium absorption. The U.S. is the biggest consumer of dairy products and sugar in the world and Americans have the highest incidence of osteoporosis (brittle bone disease). Is this coincidence? For babies who cannot be breastfed, goat's milk provides a much more digestible alternative than cow's milk and most people with allergies to dairy foods are not allergic to goat's cheese. Over-consumption of meat and dairy products may well be one of the great causes of ill-health in the Western world.

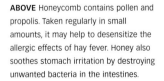

ABOVE Honeycomb contains pollen and propolis. Taken regularly in small amounts, it may help to desensitize the allergic effects of hay fever. Honey also soothes stomach irritation by destroying unwanted bacteria in the intestines.

ADDITIVES LINKED TO HEALTH PROBLEMS

	* Hyperactivity	#Asthma	+General allergies	>Not good for babies
E102 Tartrazine	*	#		
E104 Quinoline Yellow	*			
107 Yellow 2G	*			
E110 Sunset Yellow	*			
E120 Cochineal	*			
E122 Carmoisine	*	#		
E123 Amaranth	*			
E124 Ponceau 4R	*	#		
E127 Erythrosine	*			
128 Red 2G	*			
E131 Patent blue V	*	#	+	
E132 Indigo Carmine	*	#	+	
E133 Brilliant Blue	*			
E142 Green S	*			
E150 Caramel	*			
E151 Black PN	*			
E153 Carbon Black	*			
E154 Brown FK	*			
155 Brown HT	*			
E200 Sorbic acid			+	
E210 Benzoic acid	*	#	+	
E211 Sodium Benzoate	*	#	+	
E212 Potassium benzoate	*		+	
E213 Calcium benzoate	*		+	
E214-219 Hydroxy-benzoate salts	*		+	
E222 Sodium hydrogen sulfite	*			
E223 Sodium metabisulfite	*			
E224 Potassium metabisulfite	*			
E226 Calcium sulfite	*			
E227 Calcium hydrogen sulfite	*			
E249 Potassium nitrite	*	#		>
E250 Sodium nitrite	*		+	>
E251 Sodium nitrate	*		+	>
E252 Potassium nitrate	*		+	>
E270 Lactic acid				>
E310 Propylgallate,				
E311 Octyl gallate, and				
E312 Dodecyl gallate	*	#		>
E320 Butylated hydroxytoluene (BHA)	*	#	+	>
E321 Butylated hydroxytoluene (BHT)	*	#	+	>
E406 Agar			+	
E430 Poloxyethylene (8) stearate and				
E431 Polyoxyethylene stearate			+	
E508 Potassium chloride			+	
E510 Ammonium chloride			+	
514 Sodium sulfate			+	>
541 Sodium aluminum phosphate			+	>
621 Monosodium glutamate (MSG)	*	#	+	>
622 Monopotassium glutamate	*	#	+	>
627 Sodium guanylate, 631 Sodium inosinate and Sodium-5-ribonucleotide	*		+	>
924 Potassium bromate			+	
925 Chlorine			+	
926 Chlorine dioxide			+	

Additives

Additives are substances that are added to foods to help preserve them or to make them look or taste better. Some additives are natural, but a great deal are synthetic and, in the opinion of many energy healers, are at the very least unnecessary and at the worst poisonous.

Hyperactivity, asthma, irritable bowel syndrome, eczema, and other skin disorders have all been linked with intolerance to food additives.

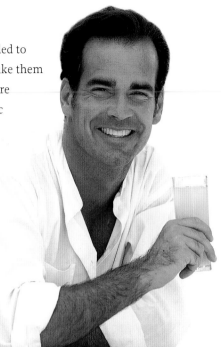

RIGHT Buy fresh, additive-free vegetable or fruit juice for a healthy, vitamin-packed drink.

Allergies

Allergies can manifest a whole host of symptoms such as asthma, eczema, wheezing, streaming eyes, rashes, and sneezing. All these symptoms are the body's way of trying to eliminate toxins (things that the biochemistry cannot deal with) from the body. Many food additives cause allergic reactions, but so too can washing powders, soaps, pollen, and animal hair. The way to cure this problem is to eliminate all artificial chemicals in your food and life, and to return to organic, natural eating. This can prove very difficult for people because the body often craves the foods it is allergic to. It can take a great deal of determination to conquer allergies but it is ultimately possible for anyone to be allergy-free.

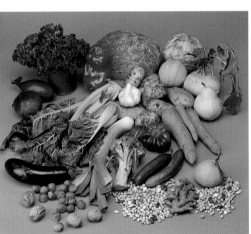

ABOVE Fresh organic food, grown without the use of chemicals, will strengthen your immune system and boost your energy levels. A totally organic diet has helped some cancer sufferers to beat the disease.

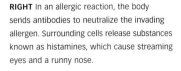

RIGHT In an allergic reaction, the body sends antibodies to neutralize the invading allergen. Surrounding cells release substances known as histamines, which cause streaming eyes and a runny nose.

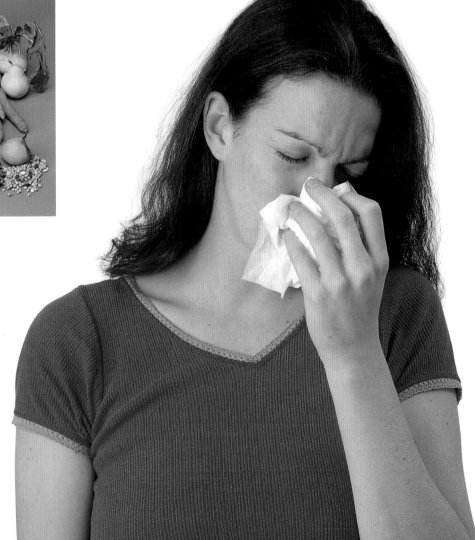

Macrobiotics and Oriental nutrition

Macrobiotics is no great secret, but it has been greatly misinterpreted and badly practiced. It has been portrayed as shallow and complex when, in fact, it is simple, but deep. Macrobiotics (macro means large, biotic means life) teaches us that food is life and that maintaining the correct balance of foods is the secret to life. But this is only one aspect of macrobiotics. Another aspect teaches that balance of the mind is also vital for health. To eat the correct foods is only half the answer. The correct food will help a person to think in a balanced way and to obtain a clear mind. In macrobiotics there is only one healer – you.

Chinese symbol of yin and yang.

Disease and degeneration recognize no boundaries. In essence, all we have to do is to employ the mind to harness the energy from the food we eat and therefore bring about the

RIGHT The macrobiotic diet is based on a balance of yin (cooling) and yang (warming) foods. Tea and coffee are extremely yin and should be avoided.

correct biochemical transformations to enable vital organ functions in the body to proceed properly. In reality, because we have become addicted to so many unbalancing foods (such as sugar, tea, coffee, and dairy products), we have lost that ability to instinctively balance our own biochemistry.

Germ theory

Since Louis Pasteur first discovered bacteria, the West has increasingly subscribed to the germ theory. This theory prescribes to the idea that germs enter the body through contamination of our foods, water, and air, or by physical contact with an infected person. It is true that certain germs can cause specific diseases, but these germs need precise conditions to prevail in order to invade the body and multiply sufficiently to cause disease. Pasteur noted in his journals that each strain of bacteria he studied required a very specific and narrow range of conditions in order to survive. These included temperature, pH balance, light, and moisture. If any of these conditions changed or were eliminated, the bacteria automatically perished. The very essence of macrobiotics is to achieve a correct balance in the body thus insuring optimum function of the vital organs and a true pH balance of the body.

Macrobiotics as the key to health

Macrobiotics has been called "a fad," "a restricting way of life," and many other things as well. In fact, it is the very opposite. It is a key to health, happiness, and fulfillment. It is not a religion nor is it a club. There is no joining fee and no badge to wear. It is a way of life based on the Oriental understanding of the laws of the universe (yin and yang). As George Ohsawa (the founder of modern-day macrobiotics) said, "There are many keys and many doors to be opened" and food is but the first. Macrobiotics insists that you take responsibility for yourself, leaving you free from debt to anyone or anything including food. It can be said that a person who eats freely but with clear thought is more

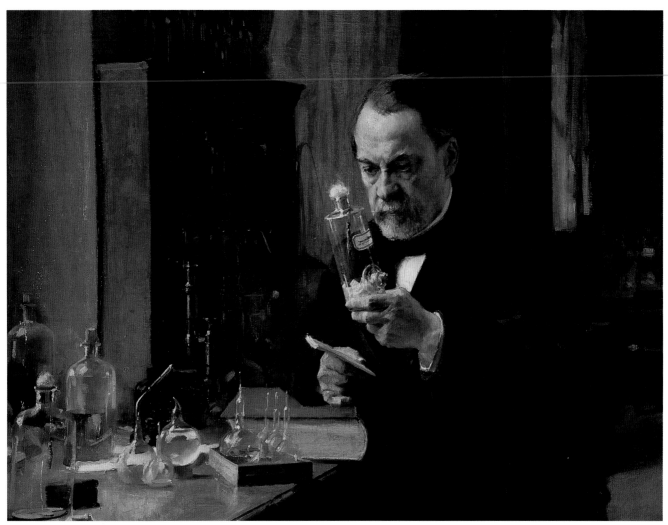

macrobiotic than a person who restricts him- or herself to brown rice and vegetables but thinks unhealthily. Driving a car requires far more skills than just steering and, likewise, macrobiotics requires more thought than just eating brown rice.

ABOVE The theories of the 19th-century French chemist, Louis Pasteur, about the spread of microorganisms led to the successful treatment of diseases such as cholera and diptheria.

LEFT The dairy products that form a large part of the Western diet are mucus-forming foods which cause an imbalance if eaten in excess.

Macrobiotic help for diseases

In the West we are plagued by an ever increasing number of diseases such as cancer, heart disease, high blood pressure, ME, irritable bowel syndrome, etc. – the list goes on and on. We are taught to view these illnesses as far too complex to understand and that we should leave the treatment of these to the professionals. These professionals ask, "What kind of disease has this person got?" while macrobiotics asks, "What kind of person has this disease?" The imbalance within the sick person's body has been brought about by their own unbalanced thoughts. This does not mean that they are insane, only that they are not thinking clearly. The mind is the host, and the body the guest.

Everything that happens in the body is but a manifestation of the mind. Dealing with symptoms through drugs and surgery is like trying to put out a fire that stems from a gushing gasoline pump by merely mopping up the spilled gasoline. Eventually you find yourself cut off and surrounded by fire. By removing the symptoms of disease, you remove the very indicators that all is not well and you walk headlong into the abyss of illness, unhappiness, and despair.

Once you understand the simple laws of nature, you realize that you shouldn't eat certain foods because eating them breaks these laws. For instance, in a cold (very yin) climate it is natural to eat red meat (very yang) frequently. In a temperate climate however, which is much less yin, eating excessive amounts of red meat causes imbalance and ill health. Likewise, in a very hot climate (very yang) it is natural to eat tropical fruits (very yin). The tropical fruits contain chemicals that cool the body down. Eat tropical fruit during winter in a temperate climate and you will over-cool the body, making it much more susceptible to attack from germs.

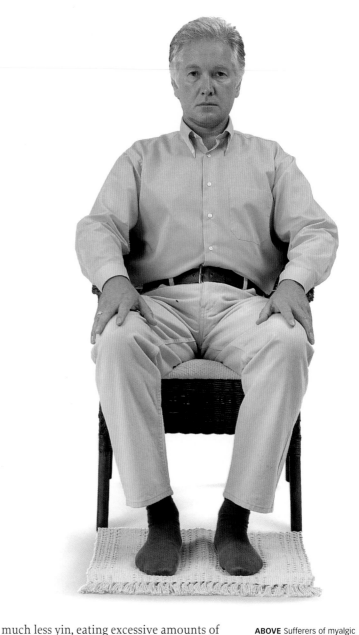

ABOVE Sufferers of myalgic encephalomyelitis (ME) experience very low energy levels and extreme fatigue. Doctors recommend a whole-food, additive-free diet in order to help combat the symptoms.

LEFT The pawpaw is a cooling fruit and an excellent source of vitamin C and beta carotene but should only be eaten in tropical climates. It also contains the pain-relieving enzyme, papain.

Ultimately, though, we should not blame food for causing our imbalance, we should look to ourselves. By allowing ourselves to be enticed by our senses and desires, we ignore the very simple and uncomplicated reasons for avoiding unnatural foods. Our minds have become latent, pushed out of the way by our senses and desire. We no longer think clearly, we no longer know our own bodies, and we no longer follow the simple laws of the universe as our ancestors did.

The true essence of a macrobiotic diet is not the eating of this or that food, it is just a discipline to help us find ourselves again. Macrobiotics offers us a chance to be free. Misinterpretation of the macrobiotic philosophy and its practice confines us to a life of narrow-mindedness.

Embarking on a macrobiotic life

The interest and acceptance of macrobiotics as a powerful, self-help therapy is growing both in North America and Europe. There are now macrobiotic societies in most countries and books on the subject, once out of print, are becoming available again.

Before you embark on "a macrobiotic life," think, think, and then think some more. Keep your thoughts simple and clear, but think deeply. If you are healthy and happy, then you will automatically be fulfilled. This is what macrobiotics offers you, but it must be done for you and by you only. In this way you incur no debt. The only responsibility is to yourself. In a disordered mind, as in a disordered body, soundness of health is impossible.

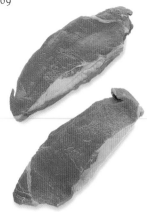

ABOVE Like dairy products, an excess of red meat causes an imbalance by heating the body.

BELOW A balanced, macrobiotic diet includes yin foods such as green vegetables, seaweed, nuts, seeds, and soybean products such as tofu (center), and yang foods such as root vegetables, whole-wheat bread and pasta, chickpeas, and brown rice.

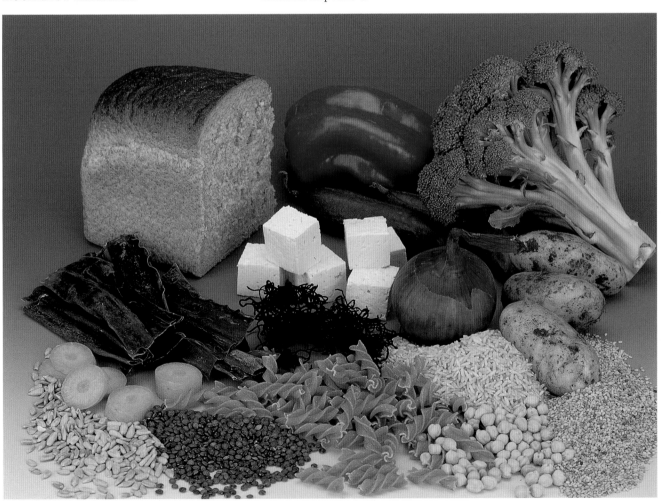

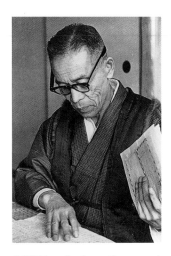

ABOVE The writer George Ohsawa cured himself of tuberculosis by using a wholefood diet that was devised by his Japanese doctor. His recovery inspired him to develop macrobiotics.

The Order of the Universe

The Order of the Universe, as taught by George Ohsawa, states that:

- Everything that has a front has a back. (This means that there are two sides to everything. There is always another perspective with which you can view things.)
- Everything that has a beginning has an end. (This means that everything has a beginning, middle, and end. Everything is a process and when you understand that process, you can flow with it instead of fighting it.)
- There is nothing identical in the universe. (This means that everything and everyone is unique and special. We all have our own talents and resources. Often we don't see them because they are masked by our imbalances in our body.)
- The bigger the front, the bigger the back. (This means that however unhappy or ill you may have felt or might be feeling, there is an equal and opposite amount of joy and satisfaction available to you if you deliberately search for it.)
- All antagonisms are complementary: i.e. beginning–end, back–front, sickness–health, unhappiness–happiness. (This means that there is always another side to life that is the opposite of what you are experiencing. You have a choice about which side you choose to live in.)
- All antagonisms can be classified in two categories, yin and yang. (Macrobiotics views the world in terms of yin and yang and seeks to find a balance between the two.)
- Yin and yang are the two arms of infinity. (This affirms the Chinese view of the universe as being made up of yin and yang in varying proportions.)

The goals of macrobiotics

- To eat natural foods. (This means whole foods free from artificial additives or other unbalancing chemicals.)
- To be free from financial worries. (This does not mean to be rich. It means to learn to not let money have power over you.)
- To achieve an instinctive capacity to avoid accidents and difficulties.
- To require no orthodox medicine or surgery. (This is a goal, not a condition. There are those foolish individuals who have turned their backs on Western medicine when they were not strong enough or wise enough to achieve this goal.)
- To live according to the order of the universe and achieve health, happiness, and freedom.

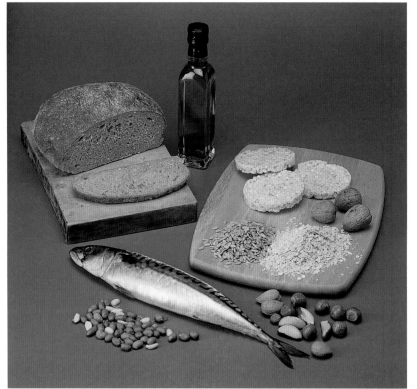

LEFT Whole grains and fish (yang) should be balanced with nuts and vegetables (yin) in the same meal. Eat no more than two small portions of fish a week.

RIGHT Macrobiotics requires a balanced approach to life. If you adopt Ohsawa's Order of the Universe, you will enjoy more energy and a healthier appearance.

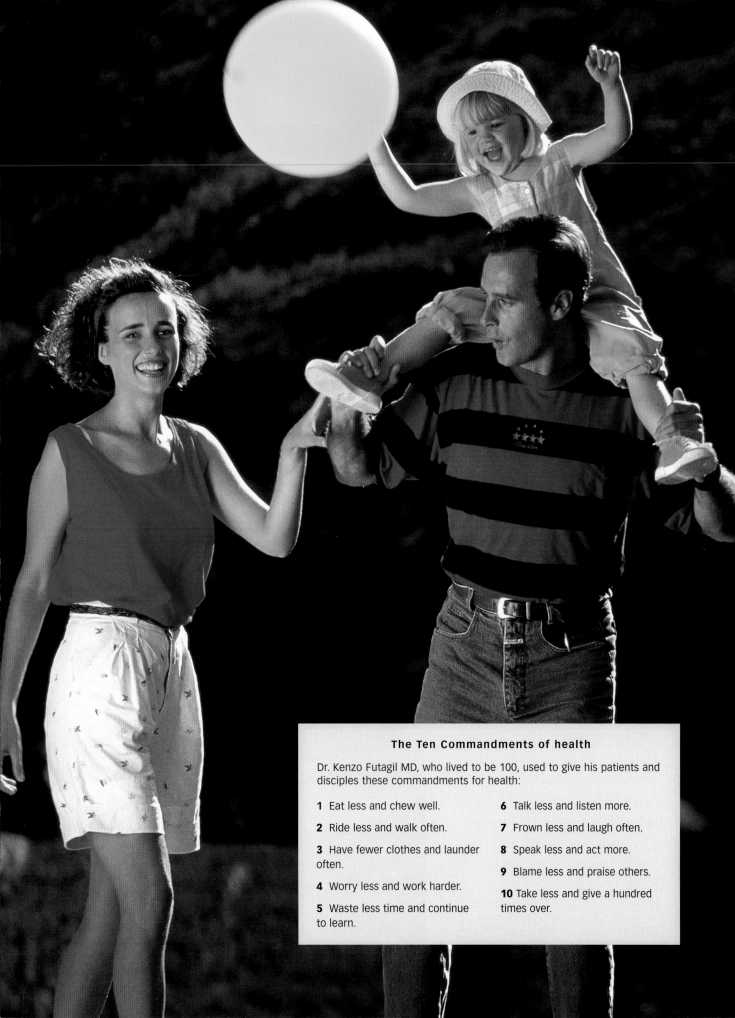

The Ten Commandments of health

Dr. Kenzo Futagil MD, who lived to be 100, used to give his patients and disciples these commandments for health:

1 Eat less and chew well.

2 Ride less and walk often.

3 Have fewer clothes and launder often.

4 Worry less and work harder.

5 Waste less time and continue to learn.

6 Talk less and listen more.

7 Frown less and laugh often.

8 Speak less and act more.

9 Blame less and praise others.

10 Take less and give a hundred times over.

Common-sense nutrition

Common-sense nutrition means thinking for yourself. You must not be fooled and deceived by the advertisements that you see every day on the news and in the streets. These are designed to lure you to buy a product that will make a company money. These companies are motivated by profit and are run by men and women who know only how to make money, and are not concerned about your health, happiness, and fulfillment.

Sadly most orthodox medical practitioners are taught very little about nutrition and can offer little in terms of sound nutritional advice. You must learn to question everything. Does a government tell you that milk is healthy and good for you because it is, or because the economic ramifications of telling the truth are too huge for any government to contemplate? Perhaps one day there will be a government or national leader who will have the vision to empower the people to make the transition from orthodox farming to farming for health. Farming organically can be equally if not more profitable than orthodox farming.

Why we need to change our eating habits

If you ask anyone if they would like the world to be a better place, they will almost certainly say yes. Well, you can make a difference right now. It takes six acres of grain to feed one acre of cattle. If we changed our eating habits and ate much less meat and many more vegetables, the world food shortage would cease to exist. On top of that, the meat you buy in grocery stores may contain antibiotic and hormone residues. Furthermore, with the inhumane

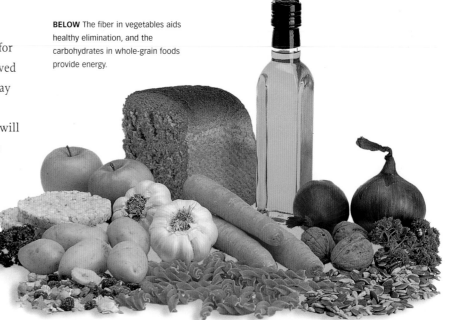

BELOW The fiber in vegetables aids healthy elimination, and the carbohydrates in whole-grain foods provide energy.

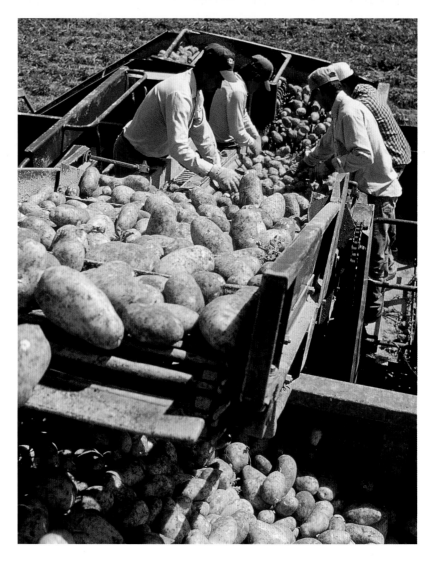

RIGHT Organic farming techniques keep the soil healthy by mixing and rotating crops, unlike modern intensive cultivation which uses chemical fertilizers to replace lost nutrients. Natural methods create produce with a better flavor.

way animals are slaughtered these days, you are also eating fear, pain, anger, and despair because they are all emotions the animal is feeling at the moment it finally dies. That negative energy is captured in the meat and released into your body when you consume it.

If you eat red meat, choose only 100 percent organic meat. It may cost more but, with all food, you get what you pay for. There is no such thing as a bargain in the food industry. If it is cheap, then the chances are it has little nutritional value and lots of harmful, but often tasty, ingredients. Stop eating for greed and start eating for health. If you do not understand these simple facts, you will never be truly happy, healthy, and fulfilled. If you spend your money on high quality, organic food and stop buying ready made, junk, or fast foods, you will find that your overall food budget changes very little.

Cook and eat only when you are in a good, happy mood. Put lots of loving, healing thoughts into your food. Stir-fry, steam or pressure-cook vegetables. Do not microwave food; cook in stainless steel or cast iron. Sit down to eat – do not eat on the move. Chew all food well. Do not drink while eating.

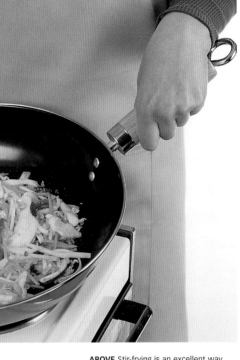

ABOVE Stir-frying is an excellent way to preserve nutrients when cooking vegetables. Warm the pan, then the oil. Add the vegetables when the oil is hot, and cook them as quickly as possible.

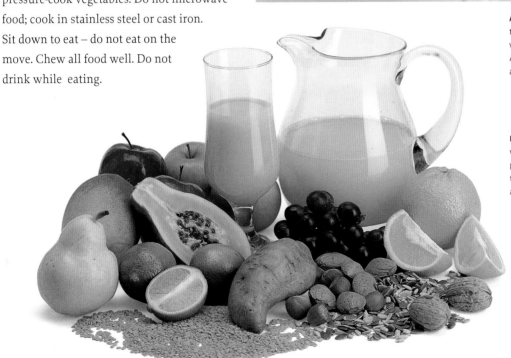

LEFT Fruit is packed with fiber and vitamins. Nuts are a good source of protein, and combined with legumes they provide a balance of essential amino acids.

Foods that are good for you

Organic white meat and deep-sea fish: Good examples are chicken, turkey, cod, haddock, tuna, hake, halibut, plaice, and monkfish.

Vegetables: Choose from the following when they are in season and locally grown – onions, carrots, parsnips, turnips, cauliflower, broccoli, leeks, scallions, radishes, beet, squash, pumpkin, beans (i.e. french and scarlet runner), vegetable marrow, celery, celeriac, watercress, sprouted beans, alfalfa, cabbage, and garlic. (Garlic is easier to digest when it has been cooked.)

Grains: Short grain organic brown rice (long grain in tropical climates) should be your staple food. Other good grains are couscous, millet, bulghur wheat, and buckwheat.

Legumes: There are plenty to choose from, such as lentils, chickpeas, lima beans, adzuki beans and mung beans.

Cereals: Oats (the best way to start your day is with porridge made with oats and water) and sugar-free organic corn (as in cornflakes).

Bread: 100 percent organic whole-wheat (unless you are intolerant to wheat or yeast, in which case try something like a sourdough rye bread).

Crackers: Rice and oatcakes provided that they are salt- and sugar-free.

Soybean products: Choose only organic, nonhydrogenated, nongenetically modified soybean products such as margarine, tofu, tempeh, miso, and soy milk.

Oils: Cook only in unrefined and cold-pressed sesame or corn oil. Use cold-pressed olive oil on salads etc.

Seeds: Eat sunflower, pumpkin, sesame, flaxseed, and pine kernels.

Foods that can make you sick

Sugar: No one should eat refined sugar. It is the hardest thing for many people to give up (it is often a hidden ingredient in foods as diverse as pizza, burgers, pastry, bread, and fruit juice drinks), but if you can do it you will ultimately realize just how energy draining and disempowering it is.

Coffee: Drink a cup of coffee after a meal and you lose 80 percent of the vitamins and minerals in that meal. You could try coffee substitutes such as dandelion or grain coffees.

Synthetic chemicals: All additives, preservatives, flavor-enhancers, and E numbers weaken and drain your energy. Many are actually poisonous to the human body.

Nonseasonal fruits: If you live in a temperate climate, tropical fruit can potentially unbalance your biochemistry. Eat only seasonal fruit and vegetables, locally grown whenever possible. Fruit should only be consumed in moderation because overconsumption can lead to the overcooling of the body, fluid retention, and hypoglycemia.

Tomatoes, peppers, eggplants, and potatoes: When eaten in excess can cause acidity in the body and are best eaten in moderation, using only organic sources. Many people are allergic to this family of vegetables (especially arthritis and rheumatism sufferers).

Seafood: Many shellfish are scavengers and because they feed off the waste and rubbish we dump into the sea, they may be filled with chemicals that can cause allergic reactions in some people.

Red meat: It takes 2–4 days to digest red meat, while it only takes 2–4 hours to digest white meat and fish. Red meat is best avoided or eaten in strict moderation.

Tap water: Filtered or bottled water is the only safe thing to drink and cook with. The chlorine added to tap water is designed to prevent typhoid, but it encourages free radical formation, which can damage cells inside body.

Dairy products: If you choose to eat them, try goat's or ewe's milk as an alternative and always buy organic.

Genetically modified organisms: No one truly knows the long-term effects of this new practice, but common sense tells you that it is unnatural to place genes from an arctic fish into a vegetable to make it frost resistant.

Chocolate: It is pure acid inside the system and, because it is highly addictive, it depletes energy and robs you of your power.

Hydrogenated fats: Hydrogenation is a process that renders vegetable oils into substances unknown in nature and which can interfere with the proper functioning of the biochemistry inside the body.

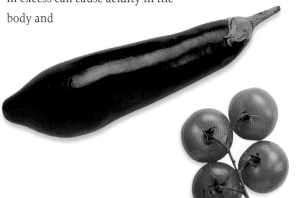

Water

There are many who advocate the drinking of a minimum of 2–4 pints (1–2 liters) of water a day. Does this really make sense? One argument is that it dilutes toxins and acid in the urine, which prevents cystitis and urinary infections, but this is treating symptoms not causes. The root causes of such problems are an imbalanced diet. Once you balance the diet, the problems disappear. Furthermore, each person's liquid requirements are different depending on their diet, lifestyle, the climate they live in, the time of year, and so on.

There is another problem: there are many foods that naturally contain water. Once it is cooked, rice is 70 percent water. Porridge also has much the same water content and the fluid content in vegetables is also very high. There are many native tribes throughout the world who get a majority of their fluid from their food. Certainly the consumption of large amounts of water has never been noted among the indigenous people of the world. Indeed the aborigines regard Westerners as being addicted to water. The only safe way to judge your liquid intake is to listen to your body and drink only when thirsty.

If you eat a balanced diet and only drink as much as it takes to quench your thirst, you should naturally regulate your water intake. Forcing yourself to drink excessive amounts of fluid is unnatural and unhealthy. A normal healthy man should urinate no more than 3–4 times in a 24-hour period and a female no more than 2–3 times. This allows the kidneys to detoxify the body efficiently.

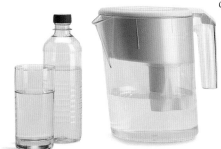

ABOVE To avoid traces of chemicals found in tap water, buy a water filter or drink bottled spring water.

BELOW Rice is a staple food for millions of people, and 90 percent of the world's supply is grown and eaten in Asia.

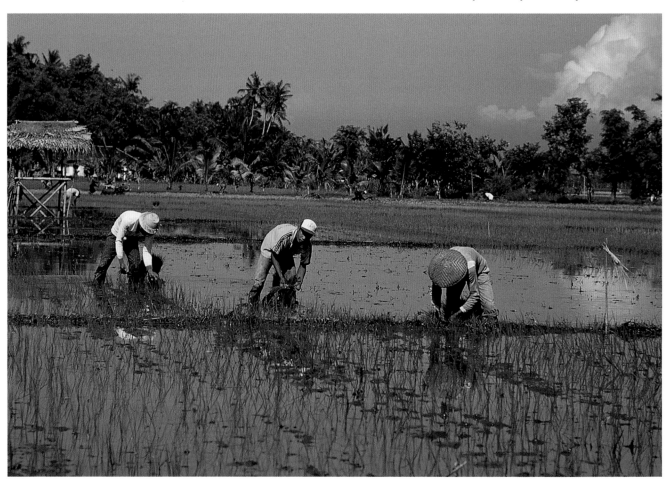

The role of the kidneys

The kidneys are the organs of detoxification. They are spongelike organs containing tiny filter tubes called nephrons. In a normal, healthy person, contaminated blood enters the kidneys and the toxins are filtered out to pass down to the bladder to be flushed away. The toxins in the urine make it dark yellow and sometimes unpleasant to smell. This is the body doing its job of elimination efficiently.

If you drink the volume of liquid that most Westerners drink and eat sugar and sweet things (which, through their metabolism, produce more water in the body), the kidneys become engorged and, as they swell, the filter tubes become constricted and you cannot detoxify. The toxins stay within the body and are stored by the liver in any available damaged or weak tissue. This is a major cause of illness in the West and is greatly misunderstood, as the following example will demonstrate: Alcohol is a diuretic, which means it takes fluid out of the body. Drinking excessive alcohol results in a hangover the symptoms of which often include a headache. This is often put down to dehydration of the brain and the person seeks to cure their headache by drinking lots of water. The standard test for dehydration is to pinch the skin on the back of your hand and then release it. If the skin returns to its normal shape quickly, you are not dehydrated. Next time you encounter someone with a hangover, try this test on him or her and you will probably find that they are not dehydrated. So what is going on?

What actually happens is that the alcohol takes the excessive fluid out of the kidneys and they return to their normal, un-swollen state. This creates the perfect environment for the body to detoxify and it begins to flood the blood with toxins to be eliminated. It is toxins in the bloodstream, not dehydration which more often than not cause the headache of a

hangover. By drinking excessive amounts of water after drinking alcohol, the kidneys swell and cannot detoxify; so the body reabsorbs the toxins and the headache disappears. But the toxins are still in the body causing potential harm. It is much healthier to simply follow your thirst and to drink no more than that.

HOW THE KIDNEYS WORK

Each kidney contains a network of blood vessels, tubes and filtering capsules. Fluid is absorbed from the blood, filtered, and excreted as urine.

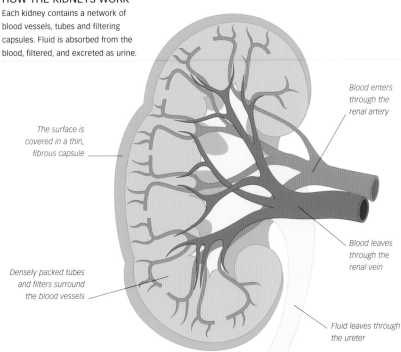

The surface is covered in a thin, fibrous capsule

Blood enters through the renal artery

Blood leaves through the renal vein

Densely packed tubes and filters surround the blood vessels

Fluid leaves through the ureter

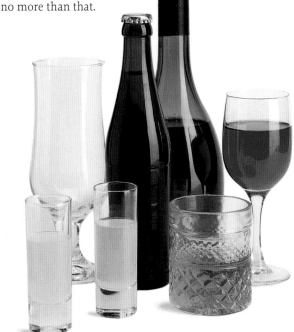

RIGHT Alcohol contains only traces of vitamins and minerals, but is loaded with calories. High intakes cause nutritional deficiencies and can have a serious effect on your health.

Hydrotherapy

Water is fundamental to all life. It is not only the major constituent of our bodies, but also the major constituent of most of our foods. Hydrotherapy – water treatment – has been used for thousands of years as a way of cleansing and healing the body. The ancient Chinese and Greeks were among the first known users of hydrotherapy. The Romans were particularly fond of it and set up baths in all the countries that they conquered. Spas and natural hot springs have always had a reputation for their healing properties and some, such as the one in Lourdes, France, have been associated with miraculous cures. Other famous towns with curative waters include Bath, Buxton, Tunbridge Wells, and Glastonbury in England, Spa in Belgium, and Baden-Baden in Germany.

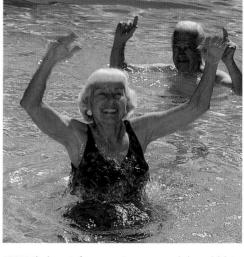

ABOVE The impact of some sports can cause pain in weak joints, especially in elderly people. Water reduces the strain by supporting the body and strengthens the muscles by providing extra resistance.

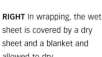

ABOVE The spa at Vichy in France surrounds a natural spring. Taking spring water to cure illness became popular in Europe in medieval times.

How hydrotherapy works

Because the body automatically responds to changes in temperature, one of the most significant factors in hydrotherapy is temperature. Hot water dilates the blood vessels, allowing warmth to penetrate and thus relax the muscles and tendons. It also promotes sweating, which is one of the body's natural detoxification processes. Cold water constricts the blood vessels, reducing surface inflammation, and promoting blood flow to the internal organs. Another important factor about water is its buoyancy. It allows the body to float and be supported without the use of muscles and this is particularly useful for those with physical handicap and mobility problems.

RIGHT In wrapping, the wet sheet is covered by a dry sheet and a blanket and allowed to dry.

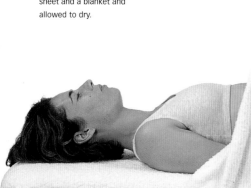

The main types of hydrotherapy

Baths: The patient is immersed in a warm bath or swimming pool to allow the relaxation and stimulation of muscles and tendons, and the release of toxins.

Wrapping: Cotton sheets are wetted with cold water and wrapped around the body to treat inflammation and skin disorders.

Compresses: Hot wraps are used to help draw toxins out of the skin.

Sitz baths: The patient sits in a tub of hot water with their feet in cold water for 3 minutes, then switches around for 1 minute. This treats constipation, cystitis, and hemorrhoids.

Steam baths: Turkish baths, saunas, and steam rooms are all used to relax the body and clean out toxins.

Who benefits from hydrotherapy?

Hydrotherapy has been found to be particularly beneficial in the treatment of chronic back pain, joint problems, arthritis, and rheumatism. It is an excellent therapy for the physically handicapped and sensory impaired and as a support for those recovering from serious accidents and injuries. It is also now being used for natural childbirth, because water provides a newborn baby with a less harsh environment than bright, artificial lighting, and cold air.

Finding a therapist

Most family doctors can recommend qualified hydrotherapy practitioners because many are attached to the physiotherapy departments of large hospitals. There are also private hydrotherapists and hydrotherapy now provides one of the main treatments offered at health farms. It is also a part of naturopathy treatment and is used to treat many ailments including asthma, menstrual pain, and anemia, in addition to those ailments described earlier.

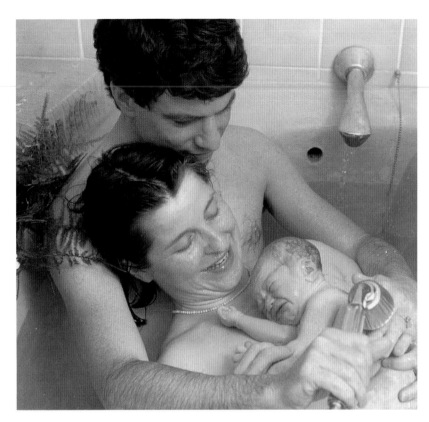

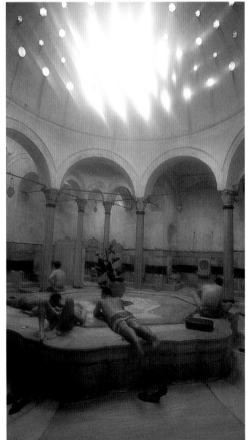

ABOVE The warmth and buoyancy provided by water helps to support the back and ease labor pains during childbirth. It can also make the birth a more natural and intimate occasion.

LEFT Humid steam rooms in Turkish baths cause profuse sweating. This removes impurities from the body, and can be used to purge substances such as drugs and anesthetics from the body. Invigorating massage is sometimes available, which speeds up the removal of toxins from the body.

Flotation therapy

Imagine floating effortlessly in a bath of water and Epsom salts heated to the same temperature as your body. With your eyes closed and with all outside stimulation cut off, you can only hear the beat of your heart and the sound of your breathing. As you become more and more relaxed, it feels as if your body and the water have become one. All the stresses of life melt away and your mind becomes still and free. It is as if you are floating in space. You feel completely safe, as if back in the womb and the boundaries of space and time no longer seem important or relevant. You emerge after what feels like 20 minutes to discover that an hour and a half have elapsed and your mind and body feel like you've just enjoyed your best night's sleep ever. This is flotation therapy.

During flotation therapy the patient lies in an enclosed tank of water, which is 10 inches (25cm) deep and filled with Epsom salts and other minerals. The water is kept at a constant 95°F (34.2° C), which is the same as skin temperature. This allows for total relaxation, and many people who experience it talk of the sensation of their bodies melting to become one with the water. A session will usually last anything from 1–2$^1/_2$ hours, although the concept of time within the tank is usually lost within the first 10 minutes of floating.

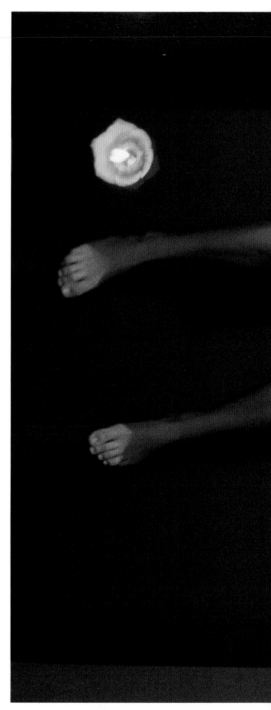

ABOVE In a flotation tank Epsom salts provide extra buoyancy, allowing the body to lie almost on the surface of the water. Epsom salts shoud not be used by those suffering from heart disease or high blood pressure.

How flotation therapy works

The flotation tank is designed to allow the patient to be in a warm, safe, enclosed environment while keeping all outside stimulation to a minimum. Sight, sound, gravity, and the presence of other people are minimized so that the patient is left alone. This creates a secure environment that facilitates deep relaxation and altered states of consciousness. During floating, the brain-wave patterns change from the normal waking beta waves to alpha and then to theta waves. Theta waves are associated with creative inspiration and deep dreaming, and often once the brain achieves theta waves the patient falls into a deep, calm, relaxed sleep. Patients can emerge

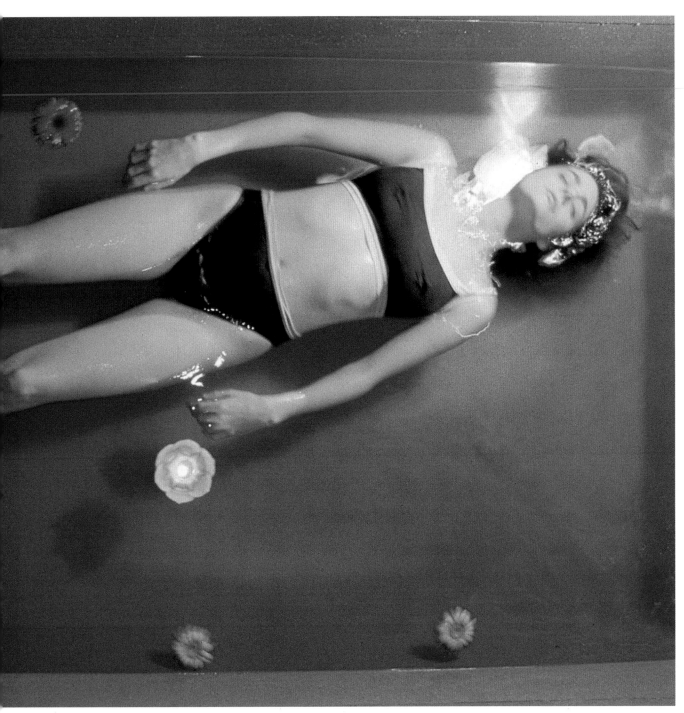

from a session with new insights and understandings of life.

Who benefits from flotation therapy?

One of the most potent effects of flotation therapy is stress relief, and so it can benefit almost anyone living in modern society. It has also proven beneficial in regulating blood pressure, helping weight loss, relieving back pain, stopping addictive behavior, improving self-confidence, increasing concentration, and accelerating learning. Flotation therapy is unsuitable for conditions such as deep depression, severe anxiety, and phobias, since it may magnify feelings of extreme negativity.

ABOVE During deep relaxation in a flotation tank, the body releases hormonelike endorphins which act as painkillers and tranquilizers. The beneficial effects of floating can last for weeks.

Energy-building exercises

Most of what we regard as exercise in the West actually uses more energy than it creates. This type of exercise is called aerobic (it uses up oxygen) and includes athletics, jogging, swimming, and dancing. All aerobic exercise is energy depleting. It burns oxygen and sugars in the body, leaving you tired and out of breath. Although this type of exercise may be good for fitness, it is not good for jing.

Energy-building exercises are anaerobic (do not use up oxygen) and not only improve the quality and free flow of chi in and around the body, they also help to build jing. All of these types of exercise are regarded as paths of learning and their practitioners are usually called masters or students. During the practice of energy-building exercises, students should keep their breathing deep and relaxed. There should be no tension anywhere in the body and, at the end of it, they should feel invigorated and completely refreshed.

Energy-building exercises can be practiced by anyone regardless of sex, age, race, religion, or position in life. Everyone can benefit from these exercises and provided they are practiced with common sense, they will not cause any harm or injury. The most important thing to remember is that all of these exercises need to be thoroughly learned and understood before safe advancement can be made. The four most common of these exercises are tai chi, chi kung, aikido, and yoga.

The benefits of energy-building exercises

All energy-building exercises are of great benefit to the body, mind, and spirit.
The body: The heart and lungs are thoroughly energized and exercised without depleting energy. The muscles, bones, nervous system, glandular system, and the respiratory, excretory, and circulatory systems are coordinated so that they all work together in harmony for the benefit of the individual. Flexibility is improved, allowing not only for freer body movement but also efficient adaptation to changes in environment. The digestive system is stimulated, allowing the efficient breakdown and assimilation of food.

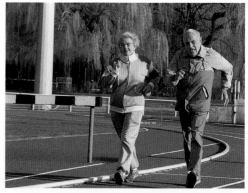

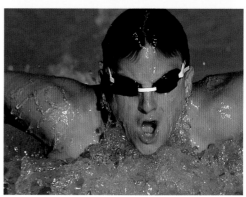

ABOVE Though aerobic exercise such as speed walking and swimming improve physical fitness, they deplete the body's energy levels and should be balanced with gentle, energy-building anaerobic exercise such as tai chi or yoga.

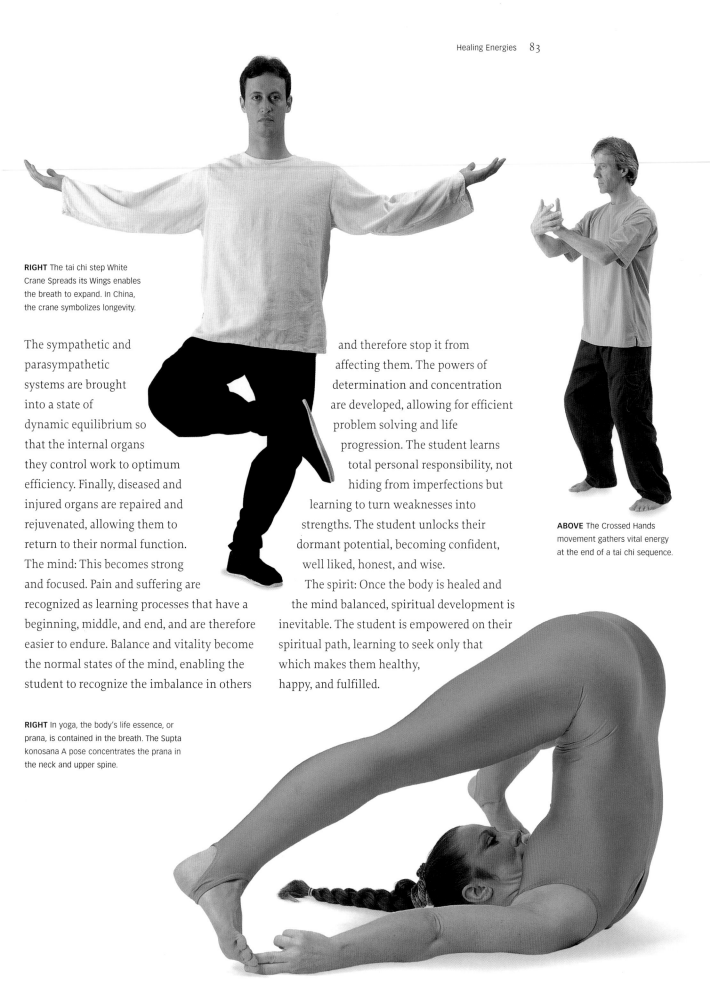

RIGHT The tai chi step White Crane Spreads its Wings enables the breath to expand. In China, the crane symbolizes longevity.

The sympathetic and parasympathetic systems are brought into a state of dynamic equilibrium so that the internal organs they control work to optimum efficiency. Finally, diseased and injured organs are repaired and rejuvenated, allowing them to return to their normal function. The mind: This becomes strong and focused. Pain and suffering are recognized as learning processes that have a beginning, middle, and end, and are therefore easier to endure. Balance and vitality become the normal states of the mind, enabling the student to recognize the imbalance in others and therefore stop it from affecting them. The powers of determination and concentration are developed, allowing for efficient problem solving and life progression. The student learns total personal responsibility, not hiding from imperfections but learning to turn weaknesses into strengths. The student unlocks their dormant potential, becoming confident, well liked, honest, and wise.

The spirit: Once the body is healed and the mind balanced, spiritual development is inevitable. The student is empowered on their spiritual path, learning to seek only that which makes them healthy, happy, and fulfilled.

ABOVE The Crossed Hands movement gathers vital energy at the end of a tai chi sequence.

RIGHT In yoga, the body's life essence, or prana, is contained in the breath. The Supta konosana A pose concentrates the prana in the neck and upper spine.

How to build energy

The four requirements for building energy are:

1 Connection to heaven and earth. For a student to successfully build energy, they must have a strong connection to both heaven and earth. This is usually achieved, initially, by the student visualizing feeling rooted in the feet while at the same time stretched upward by a silver or golden thread attached to the top of the head. As the student develops, this connectedness becomes a reality rather than a visualization and the student begins to perceive these energies working in and through them.

2 Relaxation. All muscles in the body should be in a state of relaxation. This does not mean that the muscles are not working, only that they are not tense. Tense muscles restrict the flow of blood and energy leading to tiredness and potential injury.

3 Breathing. Deep, relaxed breathing is essential for the building of energy. In the West our breathing tends to be shallow, leading to a deficiency of oxygen in our bodies. Students learn how to breathe correctly, allowing their breath to become one with the rhythm of energy pulsing around and through the body.

4 Free flow of energy. The student learns to control and direct his or her energy with the mind, thus clearing away stagnation and allowing free expression. The student learns to master their energy so that they express their lives in a healthy, happy, and fulfilled manner.

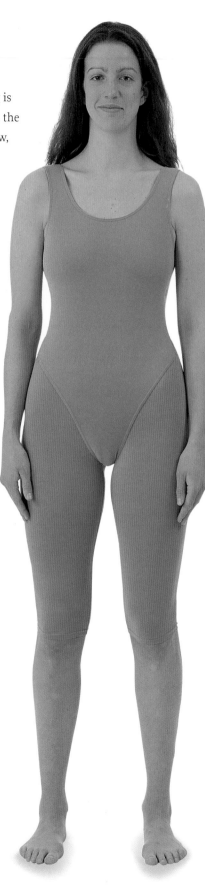

RIGHT To visualize your connection to heaven and earth, stand with your feet hip-width apart, pull back your shoulders to straighten your back and open your chest, and relax.

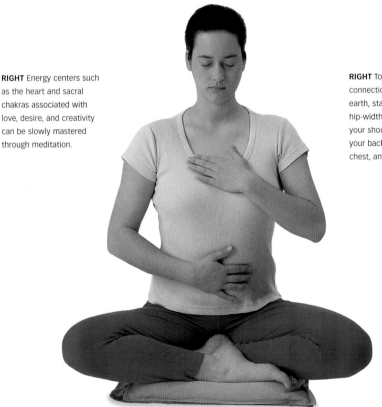

RIGHT Energy centers such as the heart and sacral chakras associated with love, desire, and creativity can be slowly mastered through meditation.

Energy-building exercise

For this simple energy-building exercise you will need a cushion to sit on and a peaceful environment to help you to relax. You may wish to play some relaxing music, burn candles and incense, dim the lighting, and unplug the telephone to help create the right atmosphere and avoid disturbance. This exercise is even more beneficial when practiced outdoors, provided the weather is fine and warm.

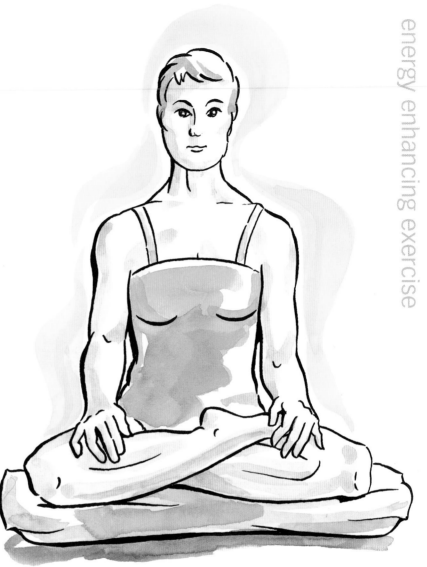

1 Sit on the cushion cross-legged or in the lotus position. Visualize roots growing from your bottom into the ground connecting you to the deepest parts of the earth. Now imagine a golden or silver thread attached to the crown of your head, pulling you upward. This should enable you to sit up with a straight back. The crown of your head is more toward the back of the head and so this should mean that your chin is inclined slightly forward.

2 Relax every muscle in your body while retaining your upright posture. Focus first on relaxing your toes, then your feet, calves, shins, knees, and thighs. Next, relax the whole of your pelvic area (hips, buttocks, and groin) before focusing on your lower, middle, and upper back, followed by your abdomen, stomach, and chest. Then focus on relaxing your fingers, wrists, forearms, elbows, upper arm, and shoulders. Next, relax your neck and face muscles, paying particular attention to relaxing every area of the face since it is often the final storehouse for our tension. Finally, relax the back and top of the head.

3 Breathe slowly and deeply in and out through the nose. The mouth should be closed with the tongue lightly resting on the roof of the mouth behind the upper front teeth. This allows the governing and conception meridians to connect, sending energy pulsing through the body.

4 Visualize your energy flowing through all your body and around your aura. Quieten your mind and try to maintain this calm, relaxed state for at least 10 minutes.

Tai chi

If you wander through any park in any major city early in the morning, you may well see a group of people performing a series of slow and graceful movements. This is tai chi, sometimes spelt taiji. Its history goes back to ancient China where it arose from combining the study of animal movements with the philosophy of yin and yang. Today it is practiced by millions of people, not just in China, but throughout the world. It can be practiced by anyone regardless of age, sex, or state of health, and its benefits are enormous and very well documented.

Tai chi comes from the ancient Chinese philosophy of Taosim, "tao" (the path) and "chi" (life energy). It consists of a series of movements called a "form." This form can take anything from 5 to 30 minutes to perform. Its purpose is to build and circulate energy around the body. In many ways it is the ultimate energy self-healing method. It has been known to help cure the incurable and in China it is routinely taught to cancer patients.

BELOW Tai chi is best performed in the open air. Its graceful movements build into one of two forms – a short sequence of about 40 moves or a long sequence of more than 100 moves.

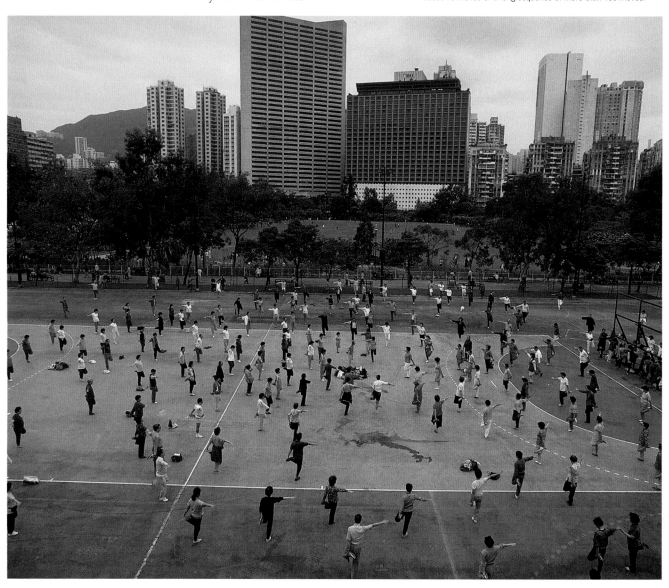

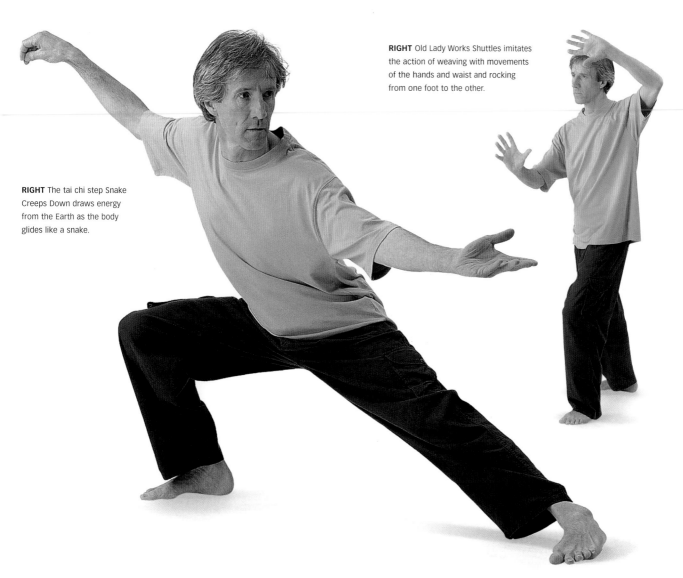

RIGHT Old Lady Works Shuttles imitates the action of weaving with movements of the hands and waist and rocking from one foot to the other.

RIGHT The tai chi step Snake Creeps Down draws energy from the Earth as the body glides like a snake.

What tai chi can do

In tai chi, improvement relies on inner awareness rather than outer strength, so it has the potential to revolutionize your whole outlook on life. If studied diligently, it will push back the boundaries of possibilities for mind, body, and spirit. It will undoubtedly improve your health and the quality of your life, and for many people it acts as a springboard into the study of many aspects of Eastern philosophy and energy healing.

Studying tai chi

There are tai chi classes in most major towns and cities throughout the Western world. There are many schools of tai chi such as yang, chan, wu, and dragon. Each has its own merits but it is more important to find a school where you feel happy and comfortable with the energy of the teacher and pupils. Most teachers will not mind you attending a class and either watching, or better still joining in, to see if it feels like the right class for you. There are many books and videos about tai chi and, though they can give you great deal of information about the subject, you will not be able to learn tai chi properly from them. If tai chi interests you, you should learn from a teacher. The learning can take anything up to a year and the greatest benefits are achieved through daily practice – the more you put into tai chi, the more you will get out.

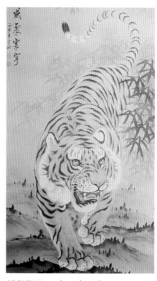

ABOVE Moves based on the characteristics of animals were developed by Taoists in the 3rd century B.C.E.

Postures

To stand with your feet a shoulder's width apart, first stand with your feet together. Turn the toes out so that the heels are at right angles to each other. Bring the heels out in line with the toes. This is a shoulder's width.

To stand with your knees bent and back straight, first stand with your heels against a flat wall and a shoulder's width apart. Pull your head up straight, slightly incline the chin forward, and bend the knees. Turn the pelvis in slightly while relaxing the lower back. If the posture is correct, only the heels should touch the wall. The buttocks and back should be clear of the wall. Maintain this position while taking two steps forward. You are now ready to begin the tai chi warm-up and walking exercises.

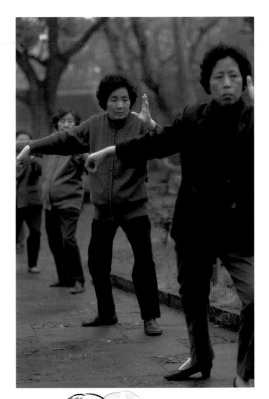

ABOVE In the basic tai chi posture, keep your center of gravity low and allow your spine to hang loose.

ABOVE RIGHT In the correct stance, the feet should be a shoulder's width apart. When one foot is in front of the other, they should follow the same line as the shoulders. The front knee should extend no further than the tip of the foot.

WARM-UP EXERCISE

This is an excellent exercise for young and old to help the body's energies to build.

1 Stand with you feet a shoulder's width apart, toes pointing forward, knees bent, and back straight.

2 Shift your weight rhythmically and slowly from foot to foot.

3 Keeping your head forward, your chin inclined, and with your eyes unfocused and relaxed, let your arms swing with the motion of your body.

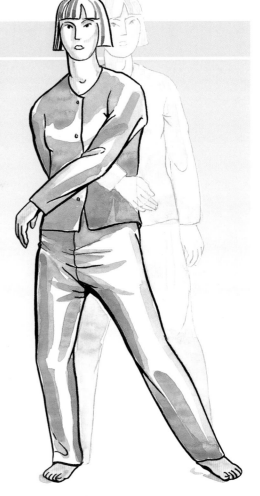

BEGINNERS' WALKING EXERCISE

While learning, all tai chi movements should be performed slowly and with grace.

1 Stand with your knees bent, back straight and feet a shoulder's width apart. Turn your left foot out to 45°. Transfer your weight slowly to the left foot and,

without leaning, lift your right foot and place it one pace forward with your foot angled at 45°.

2 Transfer the weight forward onto your right foot while maintaining an upright posture.

3 Lift your left foot and, without leaning, place it one pace forward with your foot angled at 45°.

4 Transfer your weight forward onto your left foot while maintaining an upright posture. Repeat steps 1–4.

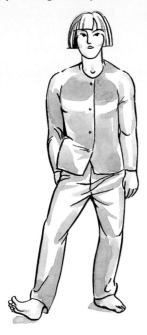
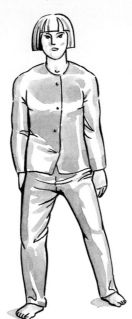
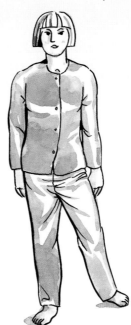
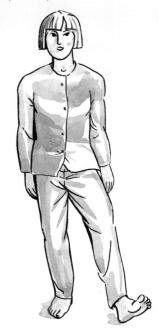

ADVANCED WALKING EXERCISE

This is the same as the beginners' walking exercise, except the arms are held up as if holding a large ball of energy. There are two positions, the arms held up (with the hands pointing to heaven) and the arms held down (with the hands pointing to earth). All postures must be maintained with the student in a state of relaxation and with normal breathing. Holding the arms aloft while tai chi walking builds large amounts of energy. Try each position for 5 minutes. You'll be surprised how hard it is at first. If you can build up to 15 minutes advanced tai chi walking every day, you will be amazed at how much energy you generate.

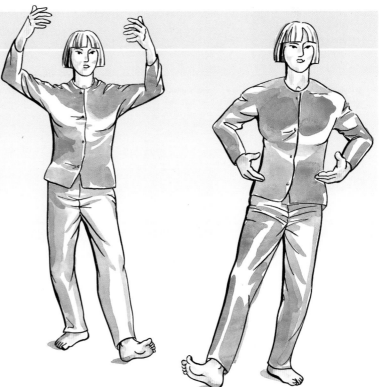

Chi kung

Chi kung, sometimes spelt qigong, is the art of cultivating internal energy (chi). The Chinese have been studying it for at least 4,000 years but until recently it was unheard of in the West. Most chi kung was kept secret, especially among the Chinese martial arts schools and religious orders of Taoism and Buddhism. Only a few acupuncturists and Chinese herbalists taught basic chi kung. Over the past 30 years however, through a new policy of informational publications and open teaching, chi kung has exploded into the West.

For the first time, health practitioners and scientists have been able to extensively test chi kung and have found it can help or cure a multitude of different diseases that Western medicine has found difficult to treat effectively, including some forms of cancer. Chi kung has been shown to help to empower individuals, turning the weak to strong, the infirm to health, and the unfulfilled to happiness. Its benefits to body, mind, and spirit are too numerous to list here but safe to say, it is of potential benefit to virtually everyone. In China it is taught as standard to many cancer patients and is now being taught to sufferers of arthritis, ME, AIDS, multiple sclerosis, and other debilitating diseases, with encouraging results. (See table on page 21.)

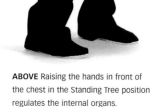

ABOVE Raising the hands in front of the chest in the Standing Tree position regulates the internal organs.

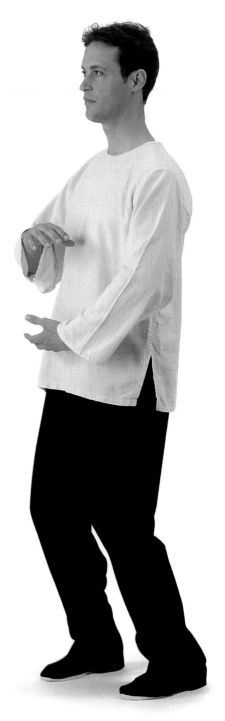

ABOVE Many chi kung steps include the pose Holding the Ball, which empowers and strengthens by concentrating the chi in the tan tien.

Chi kung masters

When chi kung is practiced as a daily discipline, tremendous amounts of energy can be built up in an individual. There are many chi kung masters in China and more are coming to the West each year. They all display exceptional energy and some even perform superhuman feats such as having a heavy truck run over then. Many of these masters are led to using their energy for healing with some very dramatic results. In China there have

even been major operations carried out using chi kung in place of acupuncture anesthesia. The chi kung master directs his energy into the acupuncture points normally used to create anesthesia. We in the West are only beginning to realize the awesome potential of chi and chi kung.

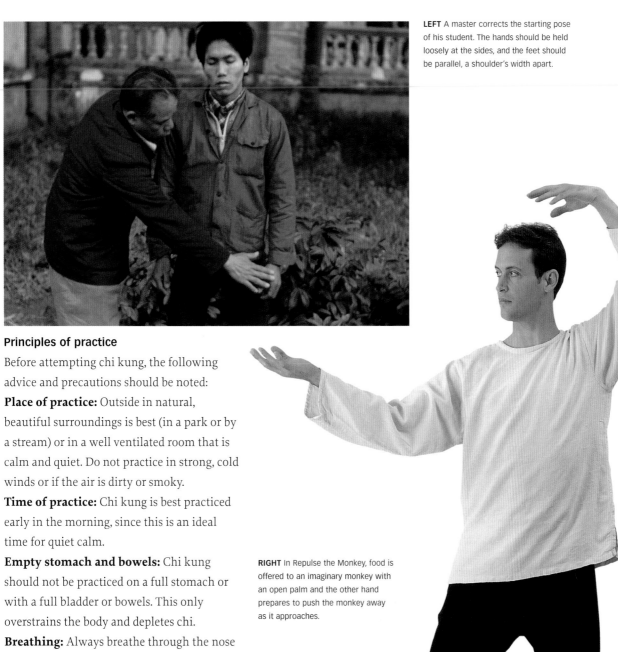

Principles of practice

Before attempting chi kung, the following advice and precautions should be noted:

Place of practice: Outside in natural, beautiful surroundings is best (in a park or by a stream) or in a well ventilated room that is calm and quiet. Do not practice in strong, cold winds or if the air is dirty or smoky.

Time of practice: Chi kung is best practiced early in the morning, since this is an ideal time for quiet calm.

Empty stomach and bowels: Chi kung should not be practiced on a full stomach or with a full bladder or bowels. This only overstrains the body and depletes chi.

Breathing: Always breathe through the nose unless otherwise instructed. Try to coordinate the breathing with the movements.

Strain: Never exert undue force or strain on your body while practicing chi kung. Although muscles are usually stiffer in the mornings, diligent practice will allow these muscles to rejuvenate to full strength without overexerting them.

Clothes: Chi kung should be practiced in loose, light, comfortable clothes. Pure silk is the preferred clothing of the Chinese.

RIGHT In Repulse the Monkey, food is offered to an imaginary monkey with an open palm and the other hand prepares to push the monkey away as it approaches.

The following five exercises relate to the five Chinese elements of metal, earth, wood, water, and fire, and their respective organs – the lungs, spleen, liver, kidneys, and heart. These chi kung exercises balance and energize all five major organs and make an excellent starting point for learning chi kung. There are six exercises in all because there is one for each kidney. Performing each exercise for 5 minutes every day will boost energy levels and strengthen the immune system.

Each exercise should be performed with slow, continuous movements in a relaxed and peaceful manner.

Lungs exercise

As you breathe in, visualize drawing pure energy into your body. As you exhale, visualize anything negative leaving and the pure energy descending to the tan tien, the spot $1\frac{1}{4}$ inches (3cm) below the navel where we store our excess chi.

Spleen exercise

Stretch your arms heavenward while relaxing your shoulders. Your hips should be pointing forward at all times: only your upper body should move.

Liver exercise

Bob up and down, keeping your posture straight and not twisting your body, while visualizing spirals of energy flowing up and down your arms and legs.

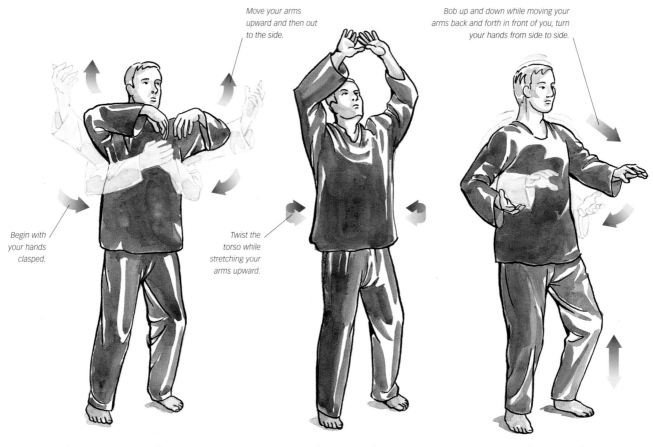

Move your arms upward and then out to the side.

Bob up and down while moving your arms back and forth in front of you, turn your hands from side to side.

Begin with your hands clasped.

Twist the torso while stretching your arms upward.

Lungs exercise   **Spleen exercise**   **Liver exercise**

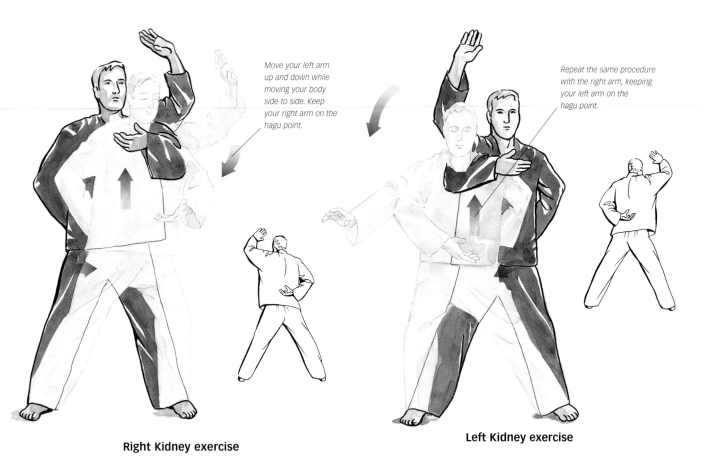

Move your left arm up and down while moving your body side to side. Keep your right arm on the hagu point.

Repeat the same procedure with the right arm, keeping your left arm on the hagu point.

Right Kidney exercise

Left Kidney exercise

Right kidney exercise

Place the acupuncture point hagu on the right hand (located between the thumb and forefinger in the webbing) over the right kidney area. Your head should be forward at all times but your eyes should follow the movement of your hand.

Left kidney exercise

Place the acupuncture point hagu on your left hand over the left kidney area.

With your hands, describe the yin/yang symbol.

Heart exercise

Heart exercise

The hands describe the tai chi symbol. Breathe out through your mouth as if you are silently sighing.

At the end of the chi kung exercises, clap your hands together and rub them vigorously until they feel warm, then wash your face three times with chi.

This helps to stop wrinkles and premature aging. Finally, draw your energies back to the tan tien three times as shown below.

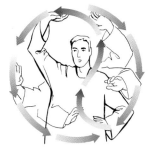

Aikido

Aikido is Japanese for "way of spiritual harmony" and describes a martial art that builds ki (chi in Chinese). Its methods resemble those of judo and jujitsu with twisting and turning techniques being used to subdue an opponent. The student learns to use his opponent's own attacking energy and turn it back on him. This means that once a student has mastered aikido, the stronger an opponent's attack, the greater his defeat.

Aikido especially emphasizes development of ki and mastery of the mind. The student learns that only by achieving complete mental calm and mastery of one's own body can one overcome an opponent's attack. The emphases in aikido are on peace and defense rather than fighting and attack. Students learn to subdue opponents, rendering them harmless rather than killing or injuring them as in some of the other, more aggressive martial arts.

The origins of aikido

The origins of aikido are unknown. It probably originated in Japan in about the 14th century, but it wasn't until the early 20th century that a Japanese martial arts master called Ueshiba Morihei developed aikido in the form we know it today. Ueshiba taught his students no attacking moves, only defensive ones and encouraged as little physical contact between students as possible. Later one of his students called Tomiki Kenji developed a competition form (known as Tomiki aikido) where one opponent holds a weapon (usually a plastic or wooden knife) and tries to score points by touching his opponent with it while his opponent tries to disarm him. The roles are then reversed.

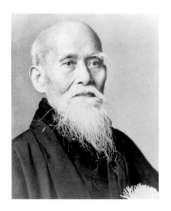

ABOVE: Aikido may have originated in Japan during the 14th century but was developed into its modern form during the 20th century by Ueshiba Morihei, the Japanese martial arts master.

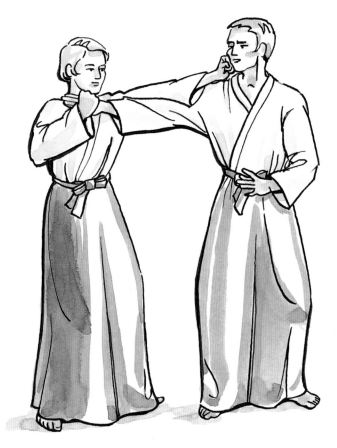

ABOVE The attacker (Uke) grasps the defender (Nage) by the shoulder. The defender turns her left hip, shoulder and foot toward her opponent. She grasps his wrist and at the same time strikes his face.

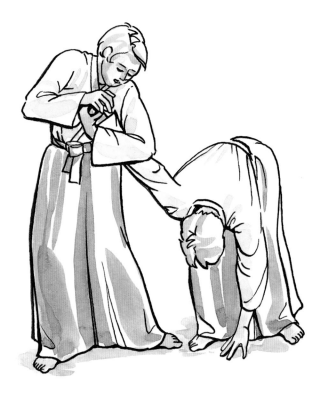

ABOVE The defender grips the attacker's wrist with her left hand, twists his hand forward and uses her elbow to push his arm forward, forcing him to bend over and lose his balance.

Finding an aikido class

Aikido, like tai chi, requires proper teaching
if it is to be fully understood and mastered.
Different teachers have different styles and it
is largely a matter of personal taste as to which
teacher you choose. An aikido teacher should
display a warm, welcoming, and totally non-
threatening energy. He or she should be happy
to talk enthusiastically about aikido and what
it means to them. Classes should have an air of
tranquility and calm about them. Aikido is an
art of expression, not aggression, and should
promote peace, not violence.

Advanced aikido teaches a variety of
pressure points on the body where vital nerve
centers exist. These points, when pressured in
the correct manner, can render an opponent
temporarily paralyzed or unconscious. There
are even points that can stop and restart the
heart. Ask the teacher whether he or she
teaches these skills. You will be able to judge
them by their answer. A responsible teacher
should never teach these skills to any but the
most advanced students who have mastered

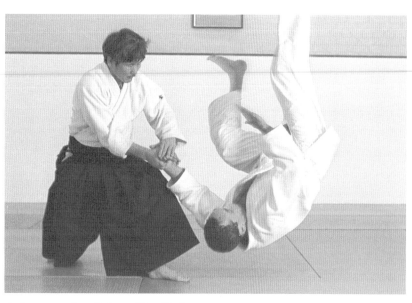

their egos and are living a life of balance, peace,
and harmony. These skills can be used to cause
great harm and a teacher who is irresponsible
with such knowledge is not a good teacher, no
matter how impressive their skills might be.

When visiting a class, sense the energy and
atmosphere. If it feels good, join. If it feels
unhealthy or threatening, walk away – it is
not the class for you.

ABOVE A participant at an aikido competition, Minoru Kanetsuke, (7 Dan) executes an outer wrist-turning throw.

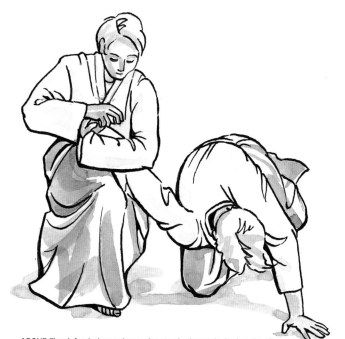

ABOVE The defender's arm keeps the attacker's arm locked at the elbow and continues to push downward, bringing his right shoulder down and forcing him to bring his right knee forward and onto the floor.

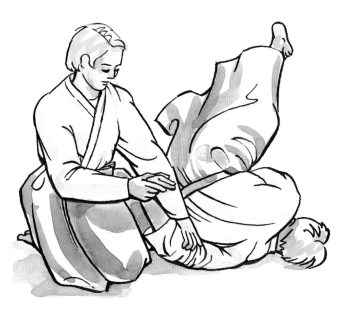

ABOVE Continuing to turn the attacker's hand forward, the defender finishes the move by pushing her opponent's elbow toward the floor with her left hand, forcing him to raise his hips and roll over to avoid injury.

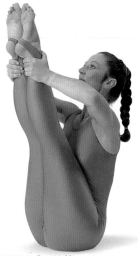

ABOVE: Urdhva Mukha Paschimottanasana pose. A balanced posture such as this requires great mental as well as physical agility.

Yoga

Over the past 20 years, the reputation of yoga as a powerful healing and rejuvenating tool for body, mind, and spirit has increased. It has been proven to be especially effective in the treatment of stress and stress-related illnesses. Recent studies have shown it to be of great help in the treatment of heart conditions, asthma, back pain, arthritis, rheumatism, anxiety, migraines, insomnia, menstrual problems, cancer, obesity, diabetes, duodenal ulcers, and addictions. Yoga teachers believe that anyone who has patience and perseverance can benefit from taking up the practice of yoga.

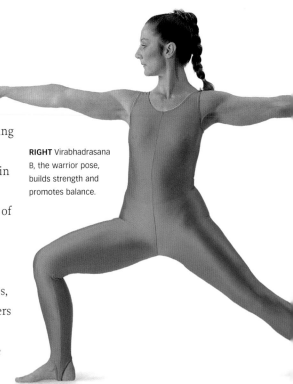

RIGHT Virabhadrasana B, the warrior pose, builds strength and promotes balance.

Yoga teaches balance of the body, mind, and spirit, and taking up yoga has for many people been a nodal point on their path to health, happiness, and fulfillment. Yoga masters display amazing, superhuman abilities such as tolerance of extreme temperatures and the ability to control the speed of the heart. Many famous and successful people accredit much of their success to the persistent practice of yoga.

The history of yoga

Like chi kung, yoga dates back at least 4,000 years. It is said to have been devised through the observation of the movements and postures of animals. In about 300 B.C.E., a yoga teacher called Patanjali divided yoga into eight classifications that are still in use today. The first two parts describe an attitude toward living. They extol the virtues of living a life of peace and harmony, following a simple diet, diligent study, and cleanliness. They warn against any form of greed and anything that causes harm to creation.

LEFT Yoga originated in India around 4,000 years ago. The practice and philosophy of yoga is devoted to balance, harmony, and inner peace in all aspects of life.

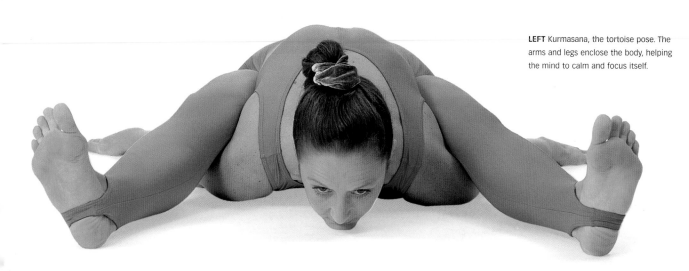

LEFT Kurmasana, the tortoise pose. The arms and legs enclose the body, helping the mind to calm and focus itself.

The next two divisions deal with the postures and their correct implementation, showing how simple exercises can calm and rejuvenate the body, mind, and spirit. The last four divisions deal with training the mind and developing spiritual qualities. They teach detachment from worldly things, acceptance of personal responsibility, mastery of the mind and body, and finally *samadhi* or enlightenment, giving the trainee deep insights into the nature of the universe.

Practicing yoga

Progress in yoga is said to come from patient, persistent practice. Finding a yoga class is a good way to learn yoga but it is only through daily practice that the benefits, such as flexibility, health, and mental clarity, can be achieved. Yoga classes should be friendly, welcoming places with a spirit of cooperation rather than competition. Classes generally last from $1-1^{1}/_{2}$ hours and most towns have beginner, intermediate, and advanced classes. Alternatively you can seek a yoga therapist who will

tailor exercises to your specific needs. The number of skilled yoga therapists is still small, as therapeutic yoga is relatively new in the West. Your physician may be able to recommend a therapist or, alternatively, most countries have yoga societies who keep registers of accredited teachers.

BELOW Urdhva Dhanuranasana, the crab pose. This posture is designed to develop spine flexibility and open the chest.

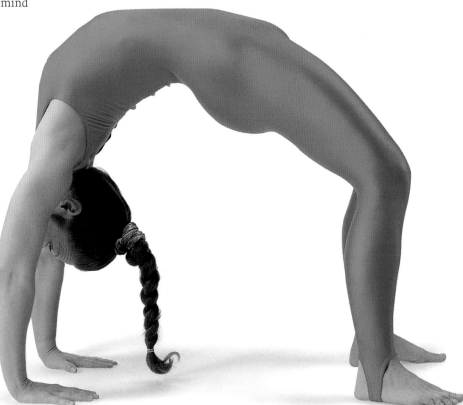

The 13 yoga postures below were designed to be performed at sunrise to help the body awaken from the previous night's rest. As they rejuvenate and energize, they can actually be performed at any time. They are quite demanding and should not be attempted (except with expert guidance) by pregnant women and those suffering from hernias, high blood pressure, or low back pain/injury.

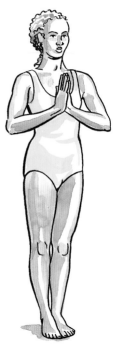

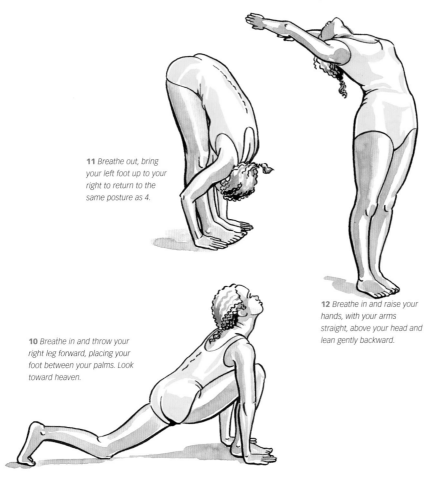

11 *Breathe out, bring your left foot up to your right to return to the same posture as 4.*

13 *Breathe out and return your palms together and against your chest.*

This is considered half a round. To complete a round, repeat the 13 postures, swapping left and right.

12 *Breathe in and raise your hands, with your arms straight, above your head and lean gently backward.*

10 *Breathe in and throw your right leg forward, placing your foot between your palms. Look toward heaven.*

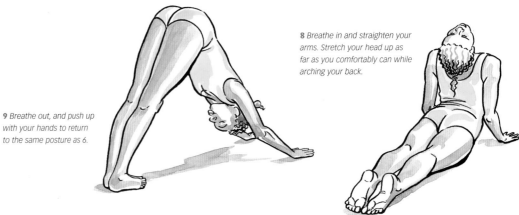

9 *Breathe out, and push up with your hands to return to the same posture as 6.*

8 *Breathe in and straighten your arms. Stretch your head up as far as you comfortably can while arching your back.*

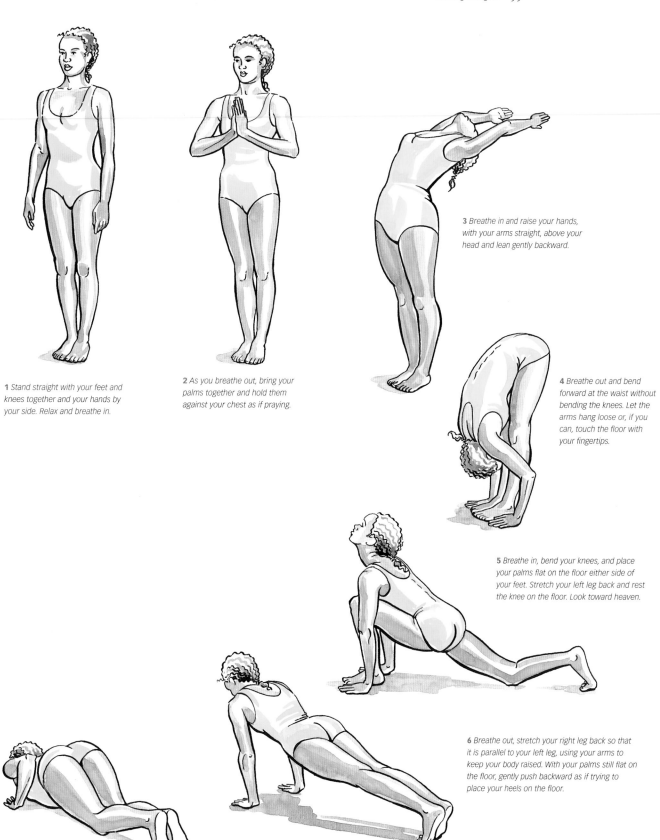

1 Stand straight with your feet and knees together and your hands by your side. Relax and breathe in.

2 As you breathe out, bring your palms together and hold them against your chest as if praying.

3 Breathe in and raise your hands, with your arms straight, above your head and lean gently backward.

4 Breathe out and bend forward at the waist without bending the knees. Let the arms hang loose or, if you can, touch the floor with your fingertips.

5 Breathe in, bend your knees, and place your palms flat on the floor either side of your feet. Stretch your left leg back and rest the knee on the floor. Look toward heaven.

6 Breathe out, stretch your right leg back so that it is parallel to your left leg, using your arms to keep your body raised. With your palms still flat on the floor, gently push backward as if trying to place your heels on the floor.

7 Holding the out breath (i.e. not breathing in), come down onto your knees, chest, and chin with your bottom raised slightly in the air.

Healing touch

"Healing touch" refers to any therapy that involves physical contact between the practitioner and the patient. There are a multitude of different techniques and therapies that can come under this banner and in many ways most of the therapies covered within this encyclopedia involve some form of healing touch. Some therapists seem to have a natural healing touch and the quality of healing does not necessarily relate to the level and complexity of the therapist's training. So what makes for high quality healing touch?

There are therapists who appear to use very few techniques and yet give high quality healing, and there are those who use a multitude of different techniques and yet get very poor results. Why is this? To understand healing touch we have to look at the five spiritual aspects mentioned in Part 1 (see page 19). High quality healing conveys high quality chen, shen, hun, po, and I from the practitioner to the patient

Chen and healing touch

High quality healing has power and this power is dependent on the level of chen in the practitioner. A good practitioner has a "groundedness" and power that they can convey to the patient. This "power" is easy to

sense because after the treatment the patient feels stronger and more powerful. If, after a treatment, you feel weak or "spaced-out" then you have not had chen transferred to you by the therapist.

Shen and healing touch

Shen is a sense of love and upliftedness. All therapists should work from a perspective of love. This means that their energy has a quality that leaves you feeling nurtured and uplifted. If, after a treatment, you feel sad or a little depressed, then you have not had shen transferred to you by the therapist. The "love" mentioned here is universal love and has nothing to do with sexual attraction and sexual energy.

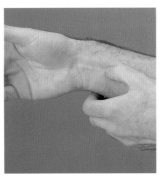

ABOVE Acupressure massages acupuncture points linked to the body's energy pathways to relieve symptoms.

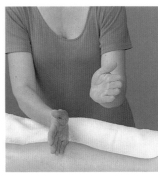

ABOVE Holistic massage compresses the muscles and lymph ducts, encouraging the body to remove toxins.

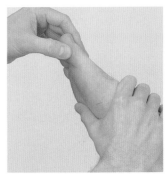

ABOVE Metamorphic technique manipulates the feet and hands to remove long-standing mental blockages.

Hun and healing touch

Hun is all about free flow of energy. All therapists should have the ability to transfer good chi to a patient but this is totally dependent on the level of hun in their own lives. Most therapists acknowledge that they are merely "channels" of healing energy, but one cannot be an effective channel if one's own energy is blocked. If, after a treatment, you do not feel energized then you have not had good hun transferred to you by the therapist.

Po and healing touch

Po is all about quality and resources. Through our interaction with others we learn new resources and improve the quality of the resources we already possess. In terms of healing touch, a good therapist should be able to transfer quality and resources into their healing. If, after a treatment, you do not feel better equipped to cope with your life, then you have not had good po transferred to you by the therapist.

I and healing touch

I is the sum total of the other four spiritual aspects. For you to receive good I from a therapist, the treatment must be powerful, uplifting, energizing, and inspiring. If you do not feel all four of these then you are not receiving good I and therefore you are not receiving high quality healing touch.

BELOW Massage brings mental as well as physical benefits. The skin contact and stroking actions soothe the nervous system, leaving the recipient reassured, calm, and relaxed.

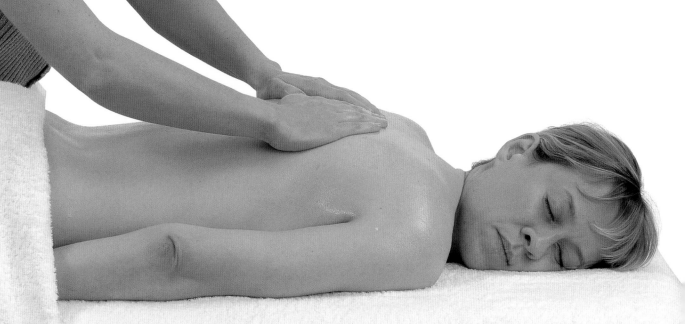

Craniosacral therapy

The cranium is the collection of bone housing the brain and is often called the skull. The sacral area of the body refers to the lower parts of the skeletal system, especially sacrum and pelvic regions. Craniosacral therapy therefore is a therapy that works on the body from top to bottom. When it first began, craniosacral therapy concentrated its treatment on the cranial and sacral regions only. Now it has been discovered that its techniques also work on the trunk, neck, and extremities too.

How craniosacral therapy works

Imagine you have a boat on one side of a canal and you want to move it to the other side. One method would be to use a pulley system to draw it across with force – this power can be likened to the strength of osteopathy. Alternatively, using just your own power, you could gently push the boat and allow its momentum to gently it across – this is closer to the light touch of craniosacral therapy. It is a subtle, yet powerful therapy that gently manipulates and balances the cranial bones, meningeal membranes, cerebrospinal fluid, intracranial vascular system, and the whole of the body's connective tissues.

A craniosacral therapist learns acute listening skills that enable him or her to perceive the subtle motions of the body. When a therapist places their hands on a patient,

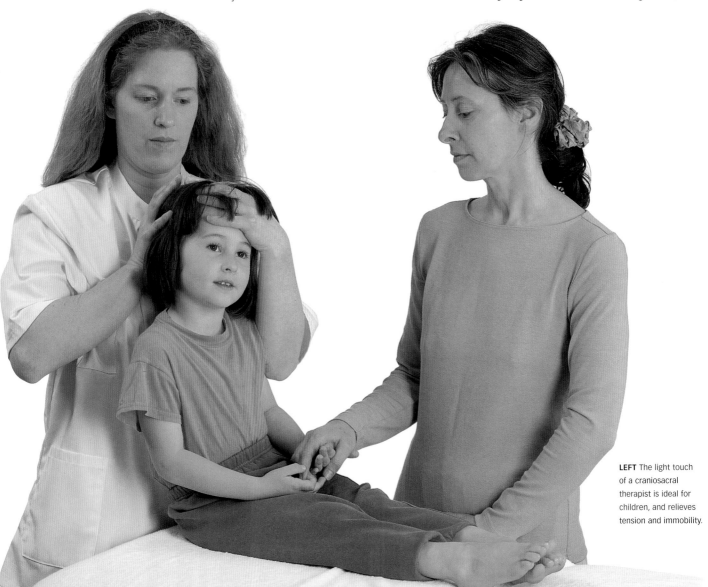

LEFT The light touch of a craniosacral therapist is ideal for children, and relieves tension and immobility.

they "listen" to the body. The body has three major rhythms. First the therapist senses the breathing of the patient. They notice this and then put it out of their minds. Then they sense the pulse of the blood flowing through the veins and arteries. They notice this too and then put it out of their minds. Then they sense the pulse of cerebrospinal fluid through the body and this is the rhythm they diagnose with. The normal rate of craniosacral rhythm (cerebrospinal fluid) in humans is between six and 12 cycles per minute. This means that the body has a subtle movement of contraction and elongation occurring every 5–10 seconds. A craniosacral therapist uses various techniques to make sure that this flow is free and balanced throughout the body.

Who benefits from craniosacral therapy?

Craniosacral therapy helps a multitude of problems and seems to produce impressive results in many cases where Western medicine can offer no cure. It is particularly useful in treating children with learning difficulties and/or behavioral problems and in treating speech problems, seizures, head injuries, obstetrical problems, ear complaints, and muscle/bone injuries.

Finding a good craniosacral therapist

Word of mouth and personal recommendation are the best ways to find a craniosacral therapist; if that is not possible, you should look for the following. A good craniosacral therapist should have trained for a minimum of two years and should hold a certificate of qualification. They should be patient and caring with a willingness to answer any questions you have about the therapy, how it works, and their personal experience of treating your particular problem. A good craniosacral treatment should give you all of the qualities described on pages 100–101.

THE STRUCTURE OF THE SKULL

The skull and the face are made up of twenty-two bones which house and protect the delicate brain and sense organs. The human skull is divided into two sections, the cranium and the face, and the only moveable bone over this surface area is that of the mandible or lower jaw.

The cranium (from the Greek word meaning helmet) comprises eight bones: the occipital bone, two parietal bones, the frontal lobe, two temporal bones, the sphenoid bone and the ethmoid bone.

The face comprises fourteen bones: two nasal bones, two superior maxilliary bones, two lachrymal bones, two malar or zygomatic (cheek)bones, two palate bones, two inferior turbinated bones, the vomer bone and the inferior maxilliary or mandible bone.

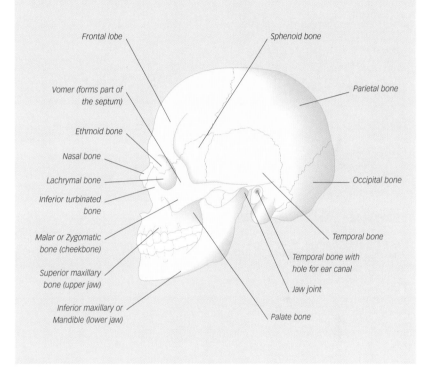

- Frontal lobe
- Sphenoid bone
- Vomer (forms part of the septum)
- Parietal bone
- Ethmoid bone
- Nasal bone
- Occipital bone
- Lachrymal bone
- Inferior turbinated bone
- Temporal bone
- Malar or Zygomatic bone (cheekbone)
- Temporal bone with hole for ear canal
- Superior maxillary bone (upper jaw)
- Jaw joint
- Inferior maxillary or Mandible (lower jaw)
- Palate bone

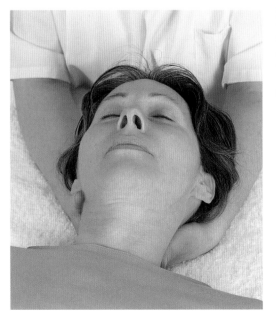

LEFT The neck also responds to the sensitive touch of a craniosacral therapist. Gentle manipulation of connecting tissues and cerebrospinal fluid corrects tiny "faults" in the alignment of the bones, which can have dramatic results.

Reiki

Reiki is fast becoming one of the most popular and widely taught therapies in the Western world. This means that there is a great

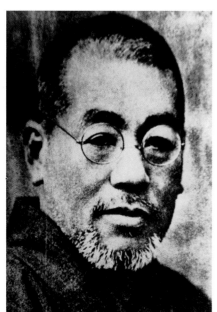

variance in quality among practitioners because although there are many excellent teachers and well-trained reiki practitioners, there are also those who have jumped on the latest New-Age bandwagon. For some, the only true qualification for calling themselves a "reiki master" is having a big enough bank balance to pay an inordinate fee for a couple of weekend workshops. Do not let this fact discourage you from discovering this powerful and potentially life-changing therapy.

Use your powers of discernment and try to follow the guidelines set out below.

Reiki comes from two Japanese words, rei and ki (loosely translated as "universal" and "energy") and is a healing system based on unconditional love. Practitioners and students learn how to tap into the healing energies of the higher spiritual planes and channel them into a patient. It is a form of "laying on of hands" but with no religion, only spirituality

ABOVE The Japanese theologist Mikao Usui discovered his ability to heal using reiki, meaning "universal life energy," after a period of intense meditation.

and love. Practitioners usually call themselves "masters." Remember, however, that the term has no real meaning and often does not indicate a formal qualification.

Who benefits from reiki?

Almost anyone can benefit from good quality reiki. It has been shown to reduce stress levels, improve circulation, and speed up healing. Many people claim dramatic improvement in a whole host of ailments and scientific research is beginning to confirm much of what practitioners of reiki have been claiming. Reiki seems to work best as a support to other therapies whether they are Western or Eastern, conventional or alternative.

Finding a good reiki master

A good reiki master is one who empowers others. They acknowledge the beauty and uniqueness of every individual and are motivated by sharing and giving rather than by money. They should be radiant with energy and full of joy. In short, they should shine with health, happiness, and fulfillment. The best way to assess a reiki practitioner, apart from admiring their shining energy, is to question them. Here is a list of possible questions that will give you an insight into

RIGHT In a reiki session, the therapist transfers their life energy to the client. In this case, concentration on the abdomen removes energy blockages and eases digestive discomfort.

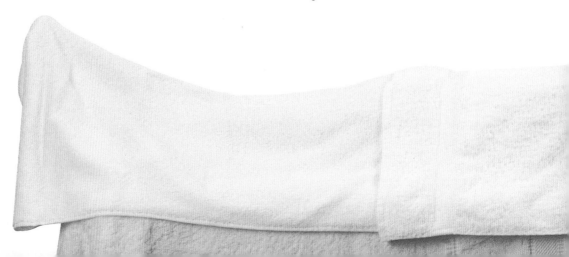

whether a reiki master is genuine or not:

1 Tell me about yourself and your background.

2 How did you come to reiki and how has it affected your life?

3 Why did you choose to become a master?

4 Are you part of a reiki organization and if so does the organization have a code of ethics that you could send me?

5 What types of illness and disharmony have you worked with, and with what results?

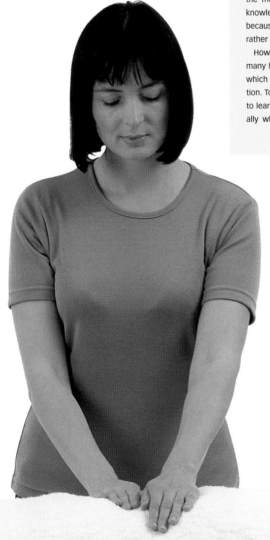

THE HISTORY OF REIKI

As a child, Dr. Mikao Usui first became inspired to heal after hearing stories of Buddha and his search for Nirvana. He was particularly interested in the tales that spoke of Buddha's ability to heal the sick. Dr. Usui concluded that there must be some truth in these ancient Buddhist stories of healing power.

He embarked on a lifelong search to discover the secrets of these special healing powers and spent many months visiting Buddhist monks in their temples the length and breadth of Japan. However, the monks that he spoke to told him that this knowledge had been lost through the centuries because they now focused on healing the spiritual rather than the physical.

However Dr. Usui was not defeated and spent many hours studying ancient Buddhist texts from which he was able to glean some useful information. To read some of these sacred tomes he had to learn Chinese and Sanskrit, and it was eventually when studying one of these ancient Indian manuscripts that he rediscovered the method of healing through using an ancient higher power.

Although Dr. Usui now possessed the written information, he did not fully understand how to use it. The story goes that he spent twenty-one days meditating on the holy mountain of Kori-yama in Japan, and on the last day he saw a beam of light on the horizon which seemed to be coming toward him. He recognized that this beam of light contained the secret of the healing power that he had hankered after for so long. When the beam reached him, he was struck on the head and rendered unconscious by the sheer force of the beam. During this unconscious state he claims to have been shown symbols which revealed to him the secrets of the Reiki healing power.

From the late 1880s onward, Dr. Usui taught reiki in Japan and trained many masters. Since his rediscovery of reiki, its popularity has spread to the Western world, and is successfully practiced worldwide by many masters and practitioners.

66 For me one of the most important aspects master (and practitioners) can bring to their students (clients) is the promotion of self-love and joy of living. In that message is also the opportunity to be of service to the people of the world. We can cocreate a peace-filled world to live in, starting with ourselves. 99

Mari Hall, International Association of Reiki.

Kinesiology

Dr. George Goodheart DC, a chiropractor, discovered applied kinesiology in 1964. He discovered that tight muscles were usually caused by weak muscles on the other side of the body. Firm massage on the ends of the muscle caused instantaneous and beneficial results. Research showed other reflexes could be used to strengthen muscles and balance organ energy, enhance blood flow, and stimulate the lymphatic system.

Kinesiology was developed for both the lay person and practitioner alike. It is easy to learn and to apply and its depth of study is dependent on what level of expertise and ability the individual wants to apply. There are various practices within kinesiology as a whole. "Touch For Health" (TFH) was designed as a basic introduction to kinesiology and "systematic kinesiology" is one of the growing fields of what is broadly termed "applied kinesiology."

Kinesiology is a form of diagnosis and therapy rolled into one. It will provide information about the patient's energy flow and offers simple but effective treatments. The basis of kinesiology hinges on simple muscle tests and using them to obtain a clear answer to a given question.

Touch For Health

TFH consists of a series of muscle tests, which shows where energy blockages are present in the body. Each energy pathway is associated with a

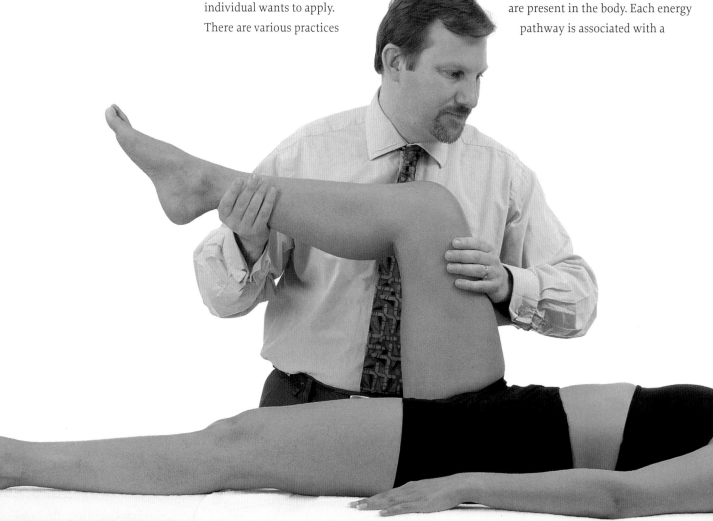

ABOVE Dr. George Goodheart founded the practice of kinesiology, which is named from the Greek word "kinesis," meaning motion.

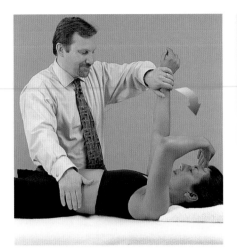

ABOVE Testing the emotional stress receptors. The arm is being pushed down and away from the patient. The patient would also be advised to avoid fatty foods, alcohol, fizzy drinks, and caffeine.

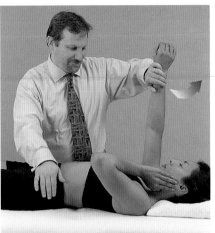

ABOVE Testing the first vertebra, which is often associated with food allergies. The patient is resisting toward the opposing hip and the arm is going back and upward. The left hand is used to check for neck problems.

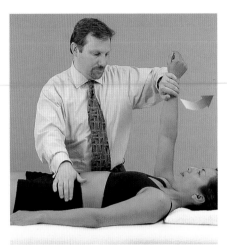

ABOVE Testing the pectoralis major sternal muscle, associated with liver problems, glaucoma, and spots in front of the eyes. The patient pushes the arm back and upward. Treatment includes massaging the chest, inside leg, ribs and under the arm. Dietary advice would include an increase in intake of foods containing vitamin A.

LEFT The therapist tests the quadriceps, pressing the knee to straighten the leg. Weaknesses in the knees can indicate problems in the small intestines. Massage treatment restores the energy flow to the muscle.

particular organ, or group of organs in the body. When testing a muscle that presents a weak response, it does not necessarily mean that the corresponding organ is weak or diseased, but is an indication that there is an energy blockage which, if not treated, could possibly lead to future problems within that area of the body.

By testing a series of muscles in the body, the practitioner seeks to find weak or strong responses. The practitioner then uses a set of readjusting techniques to fix the weak muscle tests. A weak muscle response can be strengthened by firmly massaging certain points on the body or gently massaging points on the skull. The practitioner looks for an immediate change, such as a strengthening in that particular muscle test. THF can be used in a variety of ways to aid good health, including releasing energy blockages, toning muscles, alleviating pain, and testing for allergies.

Systematic kinesiology

Systematic kinesiology uses gentle muscle tests to analyze functional imbalances in the body, then it uses touch, reflex massage, and often nutritional supplements and herbs to resolve them. The result is a speedy return to energetic health and well-being. It incorporates techniques from massage, acupuncture, chiropractic, nutrition, shiatsu, osteopathy, and others. It forms a very useful "toolkit" for practitioners of all training to use in conjunction with other skills. Used on its own or in conjunction with any type of natural health therapy, it can help relieve headaches, indigestion, stiff shoulders, anxieties, phobias, learning difficulties, backache, neck problems, and aches and pains of all sorts.

Systematic kinesiology, like all other branches of this fascinating field, is holistic, hands-on, and drug-free and may well become a standard part of all medical and alternative diagnosis and treatment.

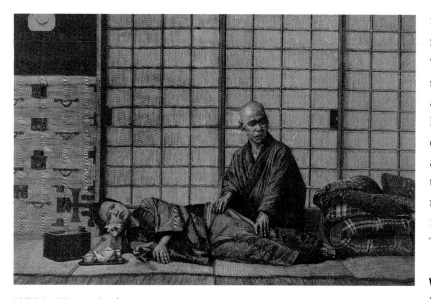

ABOVE An 1896 engraving of a Japanese masseur at work. Shiatsu stimulates electromagnetic energies in the body, balancing it evenly along the meridians, or energy pathways.

Finding a practitioner

Most countries now have accredited schools of shiatsu with registers of practitioners. Many schools offer short introductory training courses as well teaching simple and safe techniques for everyday use.

Shiatsu

Shiatsu is a Japanese word that translates as "finger pressure" although practitioners of this stimulating form of massage use the palms and heels of the hands, the forearms, elbows, knees, and feet as well as the fingers and especially the thumbs. Massage and acupressure have been practiced in Japan for thousands of years. Shiatsu has only been recognized as a specific therapy in the past 100 years. It was popularized by a man called Tokujiro Namikoshi.

Who benefits from shiatsu?

Practitioners claim that shiatsu can help a wide variety of problems including muscle and joint pain, headaches and migraines, toothache, constipation, stress, depression, and insomnia. Shiatsu is designed as a whole body therapy to stimulate circulation, and to strengthen the nervous, endocrine, and immune systems.

LEFT Before starting treatment, a shiatsu practitioner will ask you about your lifestyle and medical history, then gently feel your abdomen to assess the flow of energy inside your body.

SIMPLE SELF-HELP SHIATSU POINTS

Shiatsu massage is an easy technique to use for self-treatment. The pressure points located along the meridians are known as "tsubo," and massaging these points will stimulate a more even distribution of your body's energy.

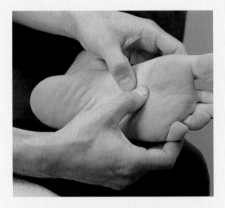

1 Press hard with both thumbs on the center of the sole of the foot for 20–30 seconds at a time to relieve dizziness and menstrual cramps. Repeat two to three times. This point is also used to treat shock, unconsciousness, and epilepsy.

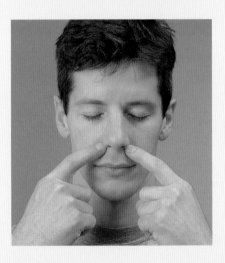

2 Apply even and firm pressure to the points under the cheekbones, below the eyes for 10–15 seconds to relieve sinus congestion, facial tension, and toothaches. Repeat twice.

3 Apply pressure with the thumb 2 inches (5cm) below the inside of the wrist. Press for 7–10 seconds, and repeat twice. This helps to ease feelings of nausea.

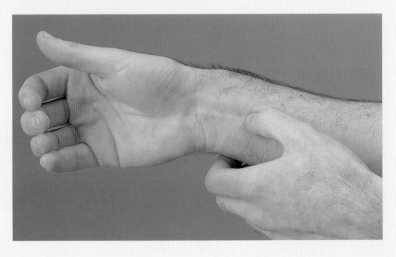

Shen tao

Shen tao is a type of acupressure and it forms a whole body therapy based on traditional Oriental medicine. It harmonizes the total being, treating deep-seated imbalances and relieving current symptoms of distress at the source. It is a subtle yet powerful therapy that activates the meridian points causing the movement and balancing of chi. This promotes deep relaxation, natural healing, and the revitalization of mind and body.

Who benefits from shen tao?

Shen tao has a remarkable ability to release many forms of stress and so it follows that any illness or condition that is directly or indirectly aggravated or caused by deep-seated stress will be soothed and healed by this therapy. It has been successful in the treatment of asthma, skin ailments, depression, digestive disorders, circulatory problems, menstrual disorders, insomnia, high blood pressure, and allergies.

The treatment

After a detailed initial consultation, a course of weekly treatments is usually prescribed. The number of treatments depends on the illness and the response to treatment varies from individual to individual. Sometimes a rapid revitalization and relief from the illness is experienced; other people with a long-standing problem may observe a steady climb back to health with a slowly increasing feeling of well-being.

Shen tao treatment is painless and usually begins with a general rebalancing of the body's electromagnetic energies. The central part of the treatment concentrates on the specific problems experienced by the patient and the session is then completed with a general balancing of the neck, shoulders, and head, which is deeply relaxing.

Metamorphic technique

Practitioners of metamorphic technique believe in a strong relationship between the foot and the body's development during the nine months in the womb. The technique was developed by a British reflexologist, Robert St. John, during the 1960s. Practitioners use gentle manipulation of the feet, hands and head to resolve and clear emotional blockages created during fetal development.

Treatment using this technique results in a change or metamorphosis of the patient's emotional state ,enabling them to become more balanced and calm.

Who benefits from metamorphic technique?

The technique is designed to help anyone with a long-standing problem, be it mental or physical. It has been of particular benefit to children and adults suffering any form of handicap and especially Down's syndrome and autism.

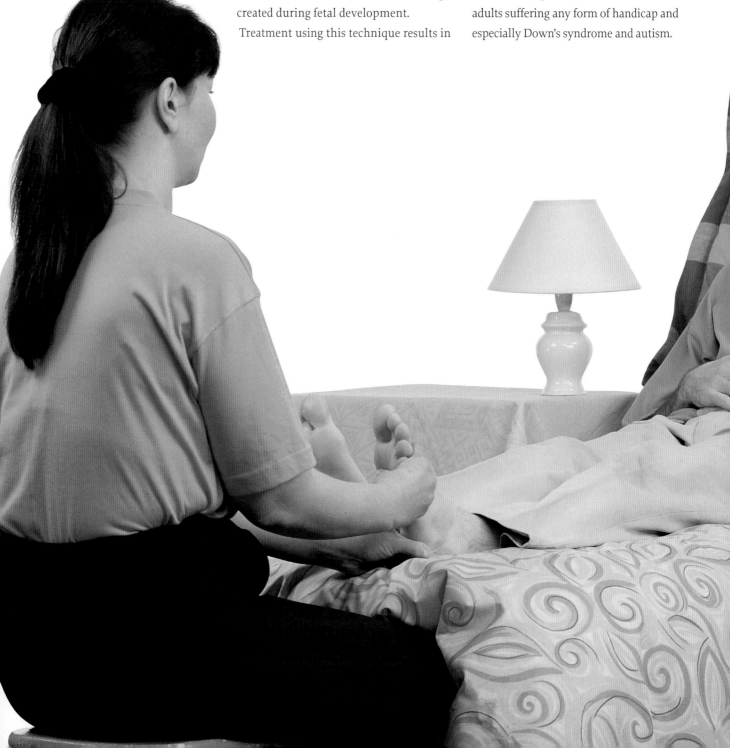

SIMPLE SELF-HELP

The best way to experience metamorphic technique is to do it yourself. There are many one- or two-day courses available and it is very easy to learn. The following is a safe and simple metamorphic treatment. It is best practiced with a friend, partner, or child and both parties are encouraged to "treat" each other.

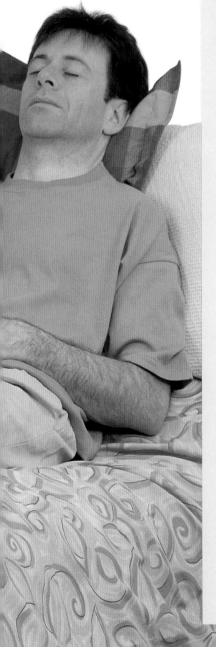

BELOW Metamorphic practitioners touch the foot lightly along an imaginary "timeline" running through the ankle and the big toe to free the client's life force and rid them of negativity carried from their past.

1. With the "patient" sitting comfortably on the floor or a sofa, take their right foot in your hands. With small, circular movements, lightly massage the ridge on the inside of the foot. Then lightly massage the entire ankle in the same way.

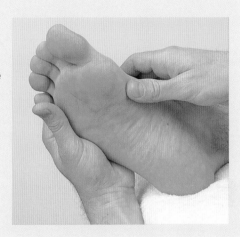

2. Now, beginning at the big toe, massage the top of the toe, then work down the ridge and around the ankle.

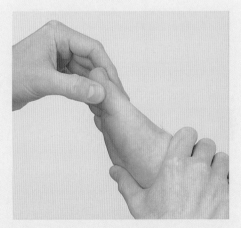

3. Repeat this movement for 10–15 minutes (5–7 minutes on a child under 12) and finish by holding the foot between the palms of your hands. Do the same treatment on the left foot for the same length of time.

During the treatment the patient may talk, sit silently, or fall asleep. When you have finished, rinse your hands under cold running water and, after a short rest, swap roles and become the patient.

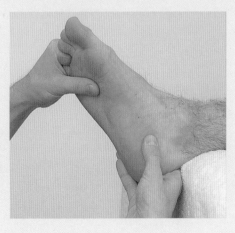

Energy massage

As its name suggests, energy massage is any form of massage that works at an energetic as well as physical level. Any massage can be "energy massage" if practiced correctly. If you have ever experienced an energy massage, you will be very aware that it is much more than just a rubdown.

For an energy massage to be effective, it needs the same four requirements as any energy-building exercise.

1 The massage must have power (chen). This does not mean it should be forceful, deep, or heavy handed. It means that the patient must feel grounded by the power of the therapist coming through the massage.

2 It must relax and uplift (shen). This can only be achieved if the therapist works from a perspective of unconditional, universal love.

3 It must improve the quality of life for both therapist and patient (po). This is achieved through deep, relaxed breathing, allowing for full oxygenation of the body.

4 It must transmit energy (hun). This is the vital ingredient in energy massage and is achieved through the therapist mastering their ego and setting forth a pure intent to allow their energy to freely flow directly into their patient.

These are the requirements of energy massage that every patient and practitioner should look for.

Polarity therapy

Dr. Randolph Stone (1890–1983) was born in Austria but trained and worked in the United States. He practiced naturopathy and the bone-manipulating therapies of osteopathy and chiropractic. He also studied many Eastern energy-healing techniques including acupuncture, Ayurvedic medicine, and yoga. From this knowledge he created polarity therapy over the course of some 50 years as a means of helping the body to balance and heal itself.

The following four techniques designed by Dr. Stone are used by polarity therapists today.

Manipulation and touch: The therapist uses his hands to release blocked energy and then "polarizes" the energy so that it flows correctly. There are three types of hand or finger pressure used by the therapist:

1 Positive pressure – this involves manipulation of various parts of the patient's body from head to toe.

2 Negative pressure – this involves deep tissue massage, which can be a little uncomfortable.

3 Neutral pressure – this involves light massage with the fingertips.

RIGHT A polarity therapist uses light "neutral" touch to release blockages and balance the energy centers of the body.

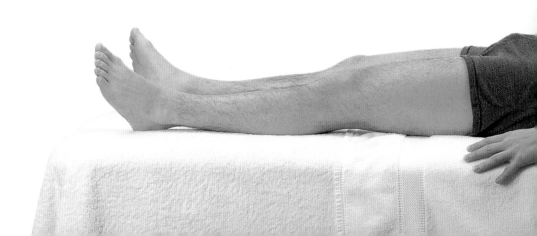

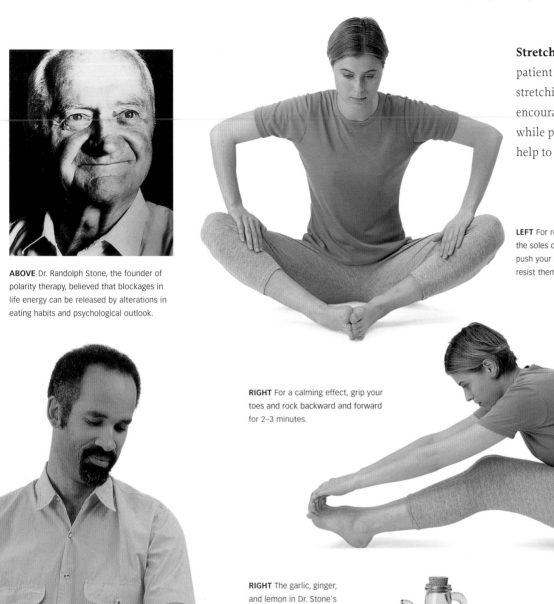

Stretching postures: The patient is taught a series of stretching exercises and encouraged to shout or groan while performing them to help to release tension.

ABOVE Dr. Randolph Stone, the founder of polarity therapy, believed that blockages in life energy can be released by alterations in eating habits and psychological outlook.

LEFT For relaxation, keeping the soles of your feet together, push your knees upward and resist them with your hands.

RIGHT For a calming effect, grip your toes and rock backward and forward for 2–3 minutes.

RIGHT The garlic, ginger, and lemon in Dr. Stone's detoxifying drink stimulate the circulation.

Diet: The patient is often put on a 14–day cleansing diet to clean the system of the toxins and impurities that can be the cause of energy imbalances and blockages. Dr. Stone invented a drink made from olive oil, lemon juice, root ginger, and garlic to help with this process.

Mental focus: The patient is taught how to change negative thinking and to open their mind to exploring new possibilities. Mental stability is fundamental to the polarity therapist's view of health.

Traditional Chinese Medicine

The roots of Traditional Chinese Medicine (TCM) go back beyond history itself. It has been practiced in excess of 3,000 years, but the exact date of its origin is unknown. The first medical textbook and the source of all Chinese medical theory is the Huang-di Nei-Ching or Inner Classic of the Yellow Emperor (hereafter referred to as the Nei-Ching). The Nei-Ching was compiled by unknown authors between 400 and 250 B.C.E. Its language is archaic and difficult to understand and so it is now usually the last text to be studied in modern schools of Chinese medicine.

In China today, the primary textbooks used to teach TCM are commentaries and interpretations of the Nei-Ching from the Ching dynasty (1644–1911). These, in turn, are modifications and reworkings of earlier commentaries from the Ming dynasty (1368–1644) right back to the Han dynasty (206 B.C.E.–C.E. 220).

Since the cultural revolution in China, TCM has spread rapidly throughout the Western world along with tai chi, chi kung, and Taoism. There are Western practitioners of Chinese herbalism and acupuncture working in most of the major towns and cities throughout the Western world. In the Chinatowns of many large cities you can find Chinese herbalists and acupuncturists who learned their craft in China and brought it with them when they traveled to the West.

The difference between Chinese and Western Medicine

At first glance the difference between Chinese and Western medical theory appears vast. Chinese medical theory does not recognize the nervous or endocrine systems and yet TCM effectively treats neurological and endocrine disorders.

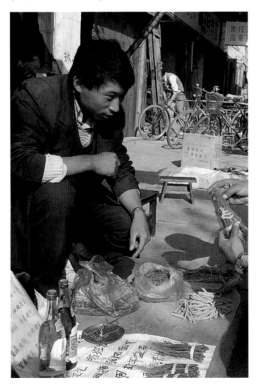

LEFT A stallholder at a Chinese market sells the cureall, ginseng, a root famed for revitalizing the nervous and immune systems and fighting fatigue. In the East, herbal self-help is a tradition stretching back for thousands of years, and the raw ingredients are easy to find.

The causes of disease according to TCM

There are three categories of causes.

External: This refers to outside factors affecting the body and includes cold, wind, heat, dryness, damp, and fire.

Internal: This refers to emotional factors and includes fear, anger, depression, anxiety, grief, and worry.

Miscellaneous: This refers to all other factors including food imbalances, physical injury, trauma, parasites, plagues, pollution, geopathic stress, "phlegm" (stagnation), and stress.

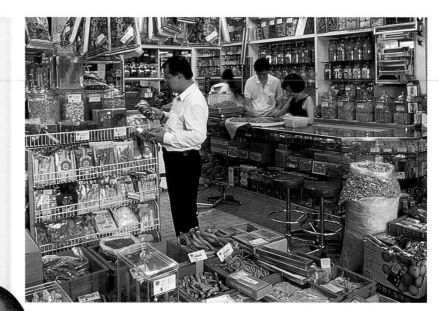

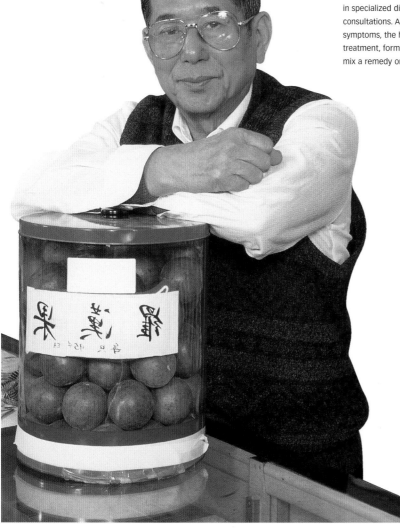

LEFT Plant medicines are not only found in the marketplace. Herbalists in specialized dispensaries offer consultations. After a discussion about symptoms, the herbalist will advise on treatment, formulate a prescription, and mix a remedy on the premises.

ABOVE The organic "herbal" ingredients and remedies that are sold in Chinese dispensaries include a few animal and mineral substances. The remedies are sold dry for making into teas or in the form of decoctions, oils, ointments, pills, and powders.

It also does not recognize bacteria and viruses as pathogenic factors and yet it effectively treats all infections and diseases. The primary difference between Chinese and Western medicine is the language and models each use to describe and treat illness and the body.

Western doctors describe the common cold as a virus attacking the body while the Chinese call it "cold and wind invading the lungs." The Chinese regard all illness as disharmony within the body and so the treatment of any illness revolves around returning the body to health and harmony. The Chinese say that it is impossible for a human whose energy is harmonious to manifest an illness. In a class of students who are all exposed to the cold virus, not every student catches a cold. Only those who have "cold and wind in their lungs" manifest symptoms. The lungs of those who remain free from illness have "harmonious energy."

Acupuncture

The first recorded therapeutic success using acupuncture dates from about 400–300 B.C.E. when a Chinese physician, Pein Chueh, revived a dying patient from a coma. It was almost certainly practiced many hundreds of years before that. In the early 19th century British doctors used acupuncture to treat pain and fevers but its use diminished with the appearance of aspirin in 1899.

Acupuncture is an ancient Chinese therapy that involves the insertion of very thin needles into the skin at specific points in order to restore the body's energy to harmony. When the cause of an illness is "Cold" invading the body, a piece of moxa (dried mugwort) is placed on the end of the needle and lit. This sends heat down the needle and into the cold area, stimulating circulation and relaxation. Moxibustion, as it is called, is particularly effective in the treatment of muscle injuries and joint pain. There are also acupuncture techniques involving the stimulation of needles with a small electrical charge (electro-acupuncture), the insertion of tiny needles in the ear (auricular acupuncture), and for those who are needle-phobic, acupuncture using lasers rather than needles.

Who benefits from acupuncture?

Acupuncture treats all manner of illness and, if professionally administered, can be more

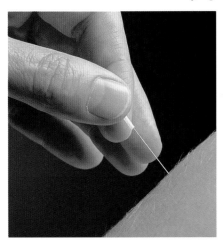

ABOVE The insertion of a fine, stainless steel needle is quick and painless. A sensation of slight numbness or tingling is sometimes felt at the acupuncture point.

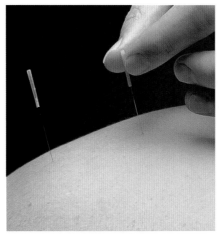

ABOVE Once inserted, the needles are left in for a few minutes to half an hour. They are rotated between the finger and thumb to draw out energy from the point.

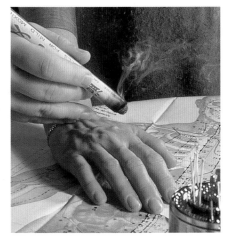

ABOVE In moxibustion, a glowing stick is repeatedly held about one inch (2.5cm) from the skin and removed when the sensation of heat becomes uncomfortable.

RIGHT A country doctor applies moxibustion to a man's back in order to warm his lungs in this painting from the Sung dynasty of 960–1279.

LEFT Moxa sticks are rolls of paper containing dried, shredded fibers of the plant *Artemisia vulgaris* (common name mugwort), also known as moxa.

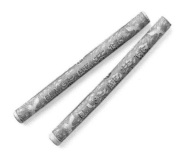

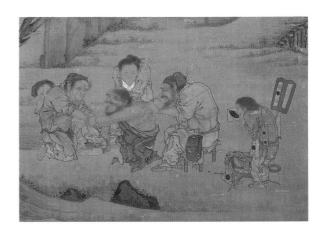

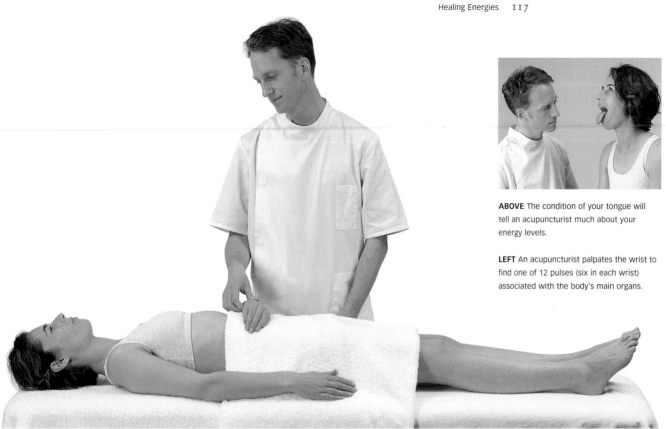

ABOVE The condition of your tongue will tell an acupuncturist much about your energy levels.

LEFT An acupuncturist palpates the wrist to find one of 12 pulses (six in each wrist) associated with the body's main organs.

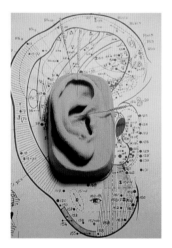

ABOVE A chart used for auricular acupuncture. The ear has more than 200 acupuncture points.

efficient at healing than many Western drugs. It is particularly useful in the treatment of pain, allergies, asthma, and other lung disorders, anxiety, neurological disorders, digestive and bowel problems, insomnia, and stress. It also works well as a supportive therapy for cancer, ME, multiple sclerosis, HIV, and AIDS.

Finding an acupuncturist

Most towns and cities have professional acupuncturists working in them, but the best way to find a good acupuncturist is by word of mouth. Classical Chinese acupuncturists tend to be very focused with their energy and this can be interpreted by Westerners as coldness or harshness. Actually they are usually very caring, it is just that their understanding of energy is far in advance of ours and they tend to be very wary of wasting chi. There are also many well-qualified Western acupuncturists if the Oriental approach is too brisk for you. Most acupuncturists now use high quality disposable stainless steel needles but if they

use reuseable needles, it is best to check that they use a sterilizing machine similar to the autoclaves that dentists use.

Consulting an acupuncturist

If you consult an acupuncturist, he or she is likely to ask you a whole host of questions about your lifestyle, diet, stress, and phobias to obtain a clear picture of your overall energy. They will then often take your pulse (pulse diagnosis is a much more complicated art in TCM than in Western medicine), look at your tongue, skin, eyes, posture, and body language to diagnose your underlying imbalances and disharmonies. They also use palpation which is a hands-on diagnostic technique involving feeling the energy flow and blockages in the body. Treatment then involves the insertion of one to 16, or occasionally more, needles for 5–30 minutes. In most cases, this process is painless. The treatment usually takes 48 hours to fully work and improvement is usually seen inside three to six treatments.

Acupressure

Acupressure, which most probably predated acupuncture in Chinese medical history, is a massage therapy involving the stimulation of acupuncture points using the fingers instead of needles. Practitioners use firm finger pressure and stimulate the points, usually for 5–15 minutes.

Acupressure is taught to all students of TCM and is also used in many other therapies including massage, shiatsu, and shen tao. It is thought that by applying stimulation to certain specific points on the body, the body's own energies are activated to help fight illness and restore harmony. Acupressure involves no equipment (the massage uses no oils) and so can be carried out in almost any situation.

Who benefits from acupressure?

Acupressure has proven particularly effective in the treatment of pain, nausea, digestive disorders, migraines, tiredness, insomnia, and depression. For many minor problems it is perfectly safe to self-administer and it is a good therapy for all lay people to gain a grounding in. There are many simple techniques that can be used for the immediate relief of minor problems, but patients who suffer from more complex complaints should consult a shiatsu or shen tao therapist.

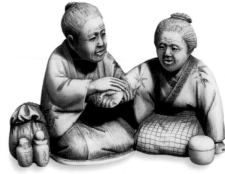

ABOVE An ivory netsuke shows a Japanese doctor using acupressure to treat a female patient.

Self-treatment

Acupressure can easily be self-administered although it is preferable if another person (a relative or friend for instance) does it. The acupuncture points used for most acupressure treatments are often slightly tender when pressure is applied to them. This makes them easy to find. Points are usually stimulated by applying pressure to the point and, while maintaining the pressure, massaging the point using rapid circular movements (60–120 times a minute). Points are usually massaged for 5–15 minutes, according to intuition, but it is worth remembering that any over-stimulation of a pressure point may well bring about a temporary worsening of symptoms.

Treating common ailments

For a headache, toothaches, dizziness, menstrual pain, and constipation, apply acupressure massage for 5–10 minutes to Large Intestine 4 (see opposite). This is located in the webbing between the thumb and the first finger with pressure directed toward the first finger. This point is nearly always tender when first massaged. THIS POINT SHOULD NOT BE PRESSURED DURING PREGNANCY. It can be used to speed up a delayed delivery, however, once labor has begun.

For nausea, morning sickness and motion sickness, apply acupressure to Pericardium 6. This point is located about 2 inches (5cm) from the inside of the wrist and

BELOW For the self-treatment of minor discomforts, acupressure is easy and convenient. Pressure points on the outside of the legs help to ease indigestion.

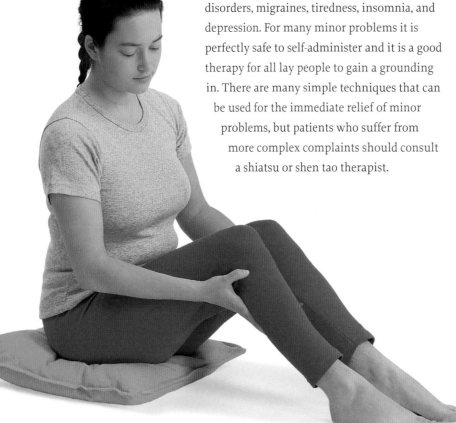
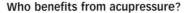

ACUPRESSURE MERIDIANS

In acupressure massage, pressure is applied to certain points along the meridians while massaging the area. Each point can help relieve specific ailments.

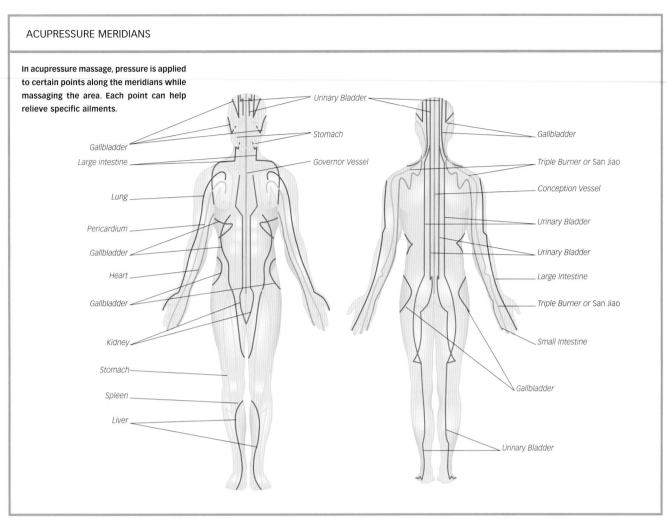

Urinary Bladder

Gallbladder

Stomach

Large intestine

Governor Vessel

Lung

Pericardium

Gallbladder

Heart

Gallbladder

Kidney

Stomach

Spleen

Liver

Gallbladder

Triple Burner or San Jiao

Conception Vessel

Urinary Bladder

Urinary Bladder

Large Intestine

Triple Burner or San Jiao

Small Intestine

Gallbladder

Urinary Bladder

should be massaged for 5–10 minutes or until the nausea/sickness subsides.

For migraines, as well as applying pressure to Colon 4, apply pressure to Liver 3, which is located in the back of the webbing between the big and second toe. Massage this point for 5–15 minutes. This point also helps to relieve stress.

For digestive disorders (diarrhea or constipation) and tiredness, apply pressure to Stomach 36, which is located about two fingers' width below the knee on the outside of the leg next to the bone. This is one of the energy-building and stomach harmonizing points used most often in acupuncture and acupressure. Massage this point for 5–15 minutes.

BELOW The web of skin between the thumb and first finger can be massaged to remove toxins and give pain relief, but should not be practiced during pregnancy.

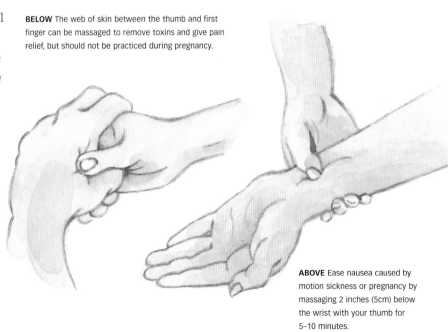

ABOVE Ease nausea caused by motion sickness or pregnancy by massaging 2 inches (5cm) below the wrist with your thumb for 5–10 minutes.

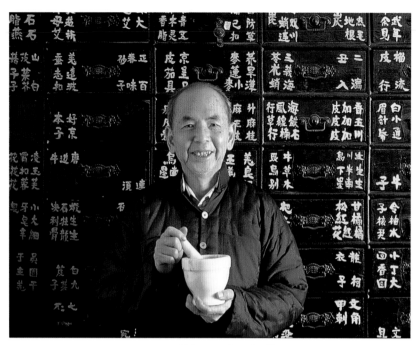

ABOVE After herbs have been cut and dried, a mortar and pestle is used to grind them into a powder for decoctions such as herbal teas.

Chinese herbalism

Over the last 5,000 years, Chinese herbalism has become established as one of the most powerful and diverse medicinal therapies in the world. Enter any Chinese herb store in any Chinatown in the world and it is like stepping back in time. The wooden drawers, the simple wooden counter, the scales, the obligatory abacus, and of course, the multitude of herbs have been part of a Chinese herbalist's equipment for the past five millennia. Chinese herbs not only consist of medicinal plants, but animal parts and minerals as well, including tortoiseshell, seahorse, lizard, and deer-horn. Illnesses are diagnosed and treated according to the five-element theory of Chinese medicine (see opposite).

Who benefits from Chinese herbalism?

Chinese herbalism treats all illnesses but is particularly effective in the treatment of eczema, asthma, digestive disorders, and any debilitating chronic illness. The herbs do not always taste pleasant but their effects are usually powerful.

Consulting a Chinese herbalist

The best place to find a Chinese herbalist is in the Chinatown of any large city. The herbalist may not speak English and may have to work through an interpreter but their diagnostic and treatment skills are usually very good. The most common prescription involves regularly drinking tea made from an herbal mixture. Recipes are usually adjusted on a weekly or fortnightly basis according to the improvement of the patient.

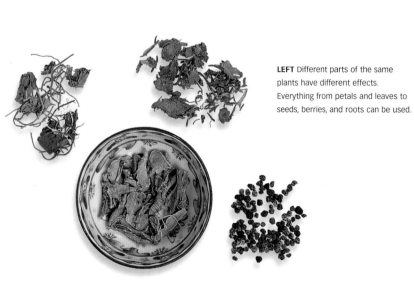

LEFT Different parts of the same plants have different effects. Everything from petals and leaves to seeds, berries, and roots can be used.

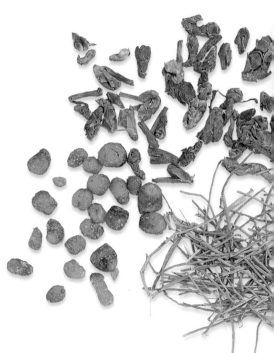

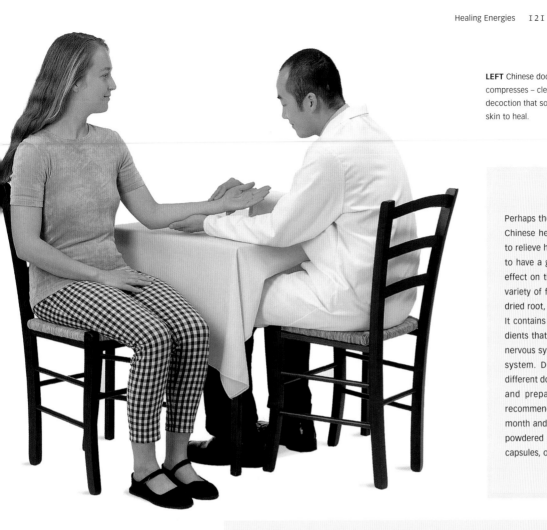

LEFT Chinese doctors often advise the use of compresses – clean cloths soaked in a hot herbal decoction that soothe inflammation and help the skin to heal.

Ginseng

Perhaps the most well-known of all the Chinese herbs is ginseng. It is claimed to relieve headaches and tiredness and to have a general tonic and energizing effect on the body. It comes in a wide variety of forms including tea, powder, dried root, tablet, extract, and tincture. It contains many complex active ingredients that are known to stimulate the nervous system and boost the immune system. Different herbalists suggest different dosages depending on the age and preparation of the plant. Most recommend a minimum course of one month and a typical dosage is 60mg of powdered root taken daily as tablets, capsules, or tea.

BELOW Up to 300 herbal remedies are used regularly. Each plant part is used in its entirety, rather than distilled, to extract the active substance.

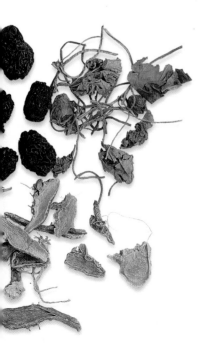

THE FIVE ELEMENTS USED IN CHINESE HERBALISM

Element	Flavor	Aroma	Related organ	Effect	Example
Metal	Hot	Rank/raw	Lungs, large intestines	Induces sweat	Fresh ginger
Earth	Sweet	Fragrant	Stomach, spleen	Digestive tonic	Chinese licorice
Wood	Sour	Pungent	Liver, gallbladder	Astringent	Sour plums
Fire	Bitter	Scorched	Heart, small intestine	Drying	Cork tree bark
Water	Salty	Rotten putrid	Kidneys, bladder	Diuretic	Seaweed

Ayurvedic medicine

Ayurvedic medicine is one of the oldest medical systems in the world. It originated in India in about 2500 B.C.E. The word "Ayurveda" comes from two Sanskrit words: ayur meaning "life" and veda meaning "knowledge" and it can be translated as "The Science of Life." Ayurveda is a truly holistic approach to healing, with prevention being at the forefront. This means that a patient is often treated before showing any major signs of illness. An Ayurvedic physician is trained in the use of diet, cooking, yoga, breath-work, meditation, and herbalism in order to restore and maintain balance in their patients.

The Ayurvedic definition of health

In Ayurvedic medicine, health is defined as soundness of the body (shrira), mind (manas), and self (atman). Each must be addressed if true health is to be attained. Ayurveda recognizes that no single agent is responsible for causing disease, but that illness is a manifestation of many levels of imbalance. Ayurveda views everything in the universe, including an individual, as being made up of three forces; vata (symbolized by air), pitta (symbolized by fire), and kapha (symbolized by water). The quality and the relative balance of these three forces are said to determine the state of a patient's health. Ayurveda also recognizes that the constitution (prakriti) of the patient can provide deep insights into the underlying causes of imbalance and disease. An Ayurvedic physician seeks to treat every patient constitutionally as a priority since it is fundamental to health and illness.

The three forces in Ayurveda

Vata is likened to the wind with its constant movement. It controls the nervous system. Vata imbalance can be caused by poor diet, irregular eating habits, or too little sleep. It manifests as any form of physical, mental, or vocal overexertion such as sudden outbursts of rage, jealousy, or an obsession with sex.

Pitta is likened to the sun, the source of energy for the earth. It controls the digestive system and all biochemical processes. Pitta imbalance is often caused by bad eating habits, leading to indigestion and acidity, manifesting as grief or fear. Alcohol abuse is also regarded as pitta imbalance.

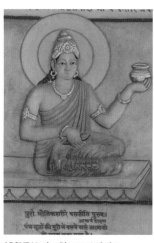

ABOVE Vasdya Dhanvantari, the supreme saint of Ayurveda, which is based on sacred Hindu writings.

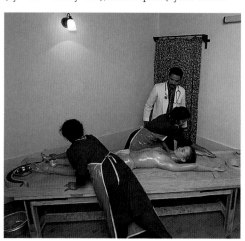

ABOVE In Ayurvedic massage, two masseurs work on either side of the body stimulating pressure points to encourage the flow of life force or prana.

Foods that benefit the three forces in Ayurveda

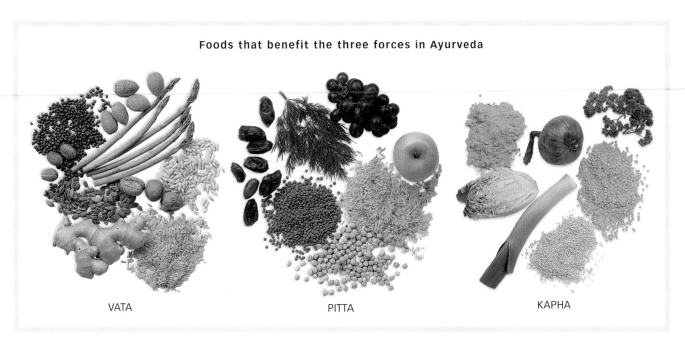

VATA   PITTA   KAPHA

Kapha is linked to the movement of all fluids in the body and to cell growth. Kapha imbalance is often caused by a lack of physical exercise or sleeping during the day. Seasonal affected disorder (SAD) is viewed in Ayurveda as a kapha imbalance.

Ayurvedic treatments

Ayurvedic treatments fall into three broad categories:

Medicinal remedies: Only natural herbs, minerals, and vegetables are used as medicinal remedies. Each patient is given a unique prescription dependent on his or her underlying imbalances. In addition, homeopathic remedies are sometime used.

Dietary regimes: As with macrobiotics, Ayurveda recognizes the importance of eating seasonally and climatically. A period of fasting is often part of the overall treatment plan.

Practical aids: These include massage, enemas, steam baths, breathing exercises, and yoga.

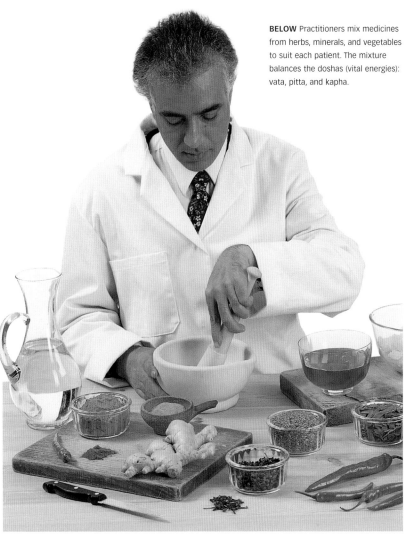

BELOW Practitioners mix medicines from herbs, minerals, and vegetables to suit each patient. The mixture balances the doshas (vital energies): vata, pitta, and kapha.

Mind energy

Eastern medicine has long recognized that the mind plays a vital role in the maintaining of health, happiness, and fulfillment. It also recognizes the power of the mind in healing. Western medicinal practitioners are now beginning to realize the same thing and "mind therapies" are becoming more widely available throughout the Western world.

All thoughts and brain waves are vibrating energy. Our brain wave patterns change according to which part of our minds we are accessing. Brain waves, like all other vibrations, are measured in hertz (Hz). There are four main types of brain waves as follows:

Beta waves: These are found in our normal waking state when our conscious mind is active. The lowest vibration of beta waves is 14 Hz with the average normal, waking vibration being at 21 Hz. A person suffering from a state of high anxiety can show a beta wave as high as 34 Hz.

Alpha waves: These occur when we are daydreaming, meditating, or in a creative state of mind. The vibration of alpha waves is 8–13 Hz and is also the normal, waking brain wave rate for animals.

Theta waves: These occur in states of deep meditation, hypnosis, trance, sleep, and shamanic activity. At this state, solid objects start to look transparent and the mind can be open to powerful levels of suggestibility. The vibration of theta waves is 4–7 Hz.

Delta waves: These occur during deep sleep but they can also occur during states of deep meditation, shamanic travel, or healing. In this state, you can no longer distinguish between the senses of sight, feeling, and sound. The dimensions of space and time become interchangeable. The vibration of delta waves is 0.5–4 Hz.

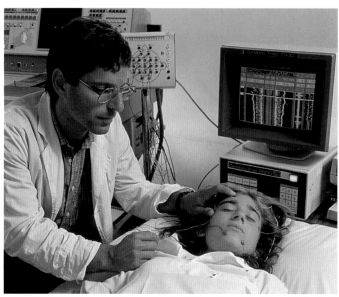

LEFT A doctor prepares a patient for an electroencephalogram (EEG), a device that records the electrical activity of the brain through electrodes attached to the skin.

The power of the mind

All illness starts in the mind. Unhealthy thinking leads to dis-ease, which manifests as illness. The mind is an amazingly powerful tool and, once harnessed, can empower you to fulfill your potential and realize your dreams. Any problem that manifests in your life is only a problem because of how you are viewing it. If you change the way you think, you can resolve anything.

The mind has the amazing ability to learn and accumulate enormous amounts of knowledge and wisdom but so often we use our minds to waste energy and to dwell on unhealthy thinking patterns that disempower us. Taoist philosophers talk of three mind states, no mind, one mind, and clear mind.

No mind state

Any thinking that is counterproductive, any negative emotions, any regret, any dwelling on the past or on possible future scenarios are all manifestations of no-mind thinking. This is how most Westerners think. We waste so much of our precious energy projecting thoughts into the past or the future instead of learning to live in the here and now. For example, if you have money problems, worrying about them will not resolve the situation. If you are in financial difficulties, the only solution lies in you actively

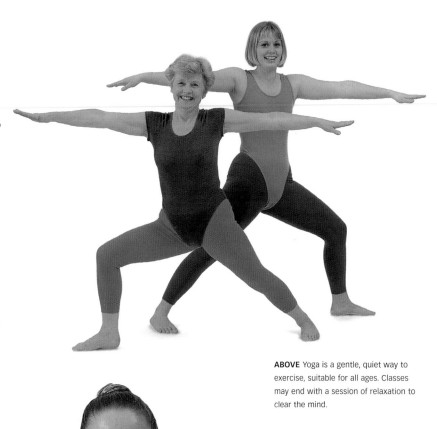

ABOVE Yoga is a gentle, quiet way to exercise, suitable for all ages. Classes may end with a session of relaxation to clear the mind.

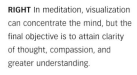

RIGHT In meditation, visualization can concentrate the mind, but the final objective is to attain clarity of thought, compassion, and greater understanding.

putting energy into your life by carrying on striving to succeed in whatever you undertake. Worrying only takes you further away from achieving this goal. Change your mind and you will realize that stressing it only serves to deplete your energy and does not help you resolve the situation.

One mind state

One-mind thinking is as unhealthy a way of thinking as the no-mind state. It is obsessive thinking that is singular and subjective. There are many people who, during their search for truth, fall into the trap of one-mind thinking. They are the sort of people who follow restrictive practices, such as special diets or hours of meditation, to such extremes that they become disconnected from society and eventually manifest illness. Any road of long-term restriction is not a road to health. We are naturally expressive creatures and long-term, restrictive practices can cause depletion of our shen, chi, and jing. This does not mean that all restriction is unhealthy. Fasting, for instance, when practiced for a short time, can be of major benefit to the mind because it sharpens and hones the senses. But any restriction taken to extremes will always lead to ill-health.

Clear-mind state

Clear-mind thinking is the type of thinking we should all strive for. The person who can think clearly is not swayed by emotions but recognizes only truth. They accept everything that comes into their lives, good and bad, and learn from it. They recognize that the past is just a memory and cannot be changed, only learned from. They recognize that the future is just a dream and that the present is the only place where they can effect change. They embrace everything with pleasure and judge no one. This is clear-mind thinking.

Harnessing the mind

The power of positive thinking should never be underestimated. You are what you think. In every situation there are positive lessons to be learned and by learning to view things from different perspectives you can greatly increase your power to learn. One of the major problems we have in the West is our inability to let go of the past. We hold onto anger and resentment, not realizing that it depletes our energy and lowers the quality of our lives. If someone is nasty to you, feeling angry toward that person takes away your power because you are allowing that person to have a negative influence on you.

A better way to handle such situations is as follows. If someone is nasty to you, recognize that you have attracted that behavior into your life in order to learn something. Rather than feeling sorry for yourself, look within yourself and ask, "What is this trying to teach me?" Once you have found the answer to that question, you will have learned something new that will have made you wiser. You can then go to the person and say, "Thank you for being nasty to me. Because of your behavior I

BELOW Emotions can often exacerbate a bad situation. Learning to let go of your need to be right will bring more harmony into your life.

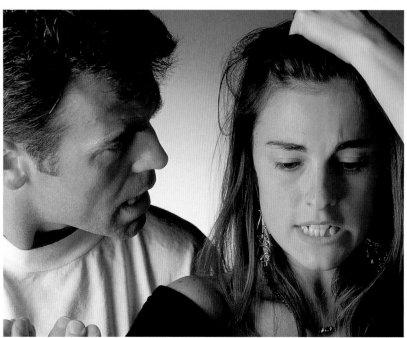

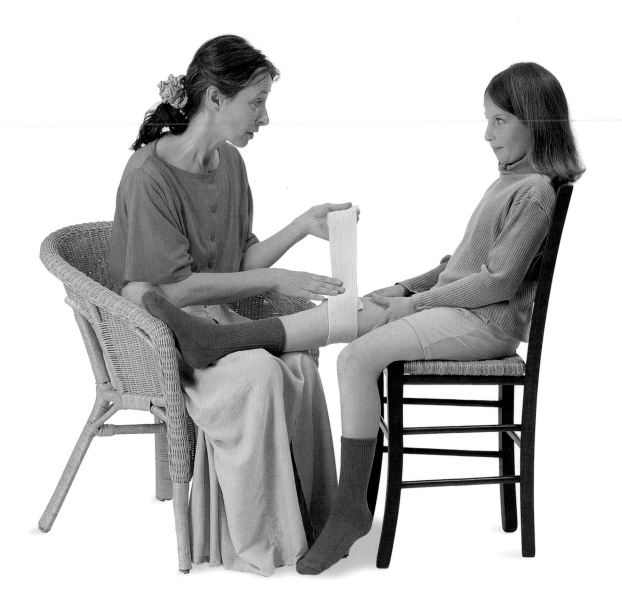

have looked deep within myself and learned an important lesson and so you have helped me to become a better and wiser person." The question of forgiveness does not even enter into things. That person has done you a favor by their actions and you can only be grateful. This is the power of changing your perspective and of turning negative into positive.

Why sympathy is bad for you

Sympathy is perhaps one of the most disempowering emotions to project toward another individual. Sympathy says, "It is alright for you to be in a negative space." Sympathy holds people in negativity and stops them from being able to turn negative to positive. If you say to someone in pain, "Poor you," you are giving them permission to carry on seeking your attention through negativity. This does not mean that you should become unemotional and detached. On the contrary, you give positive emotional energy in the form of empathy.

Empathy says, "I recognize the suffering you are experiencing at present and I want to help you to change that emotion to joy." Give empathy and support to someone in pain and you will be showing them how to change their thinking and to embrace their suffering by recognizing that it is only a learning process.

ABOVE Sympathy allows someone who is hurt to wallow in negative feelings. Compassion in the form of empathy has an uplifting effect which encourages a quicker recovery.

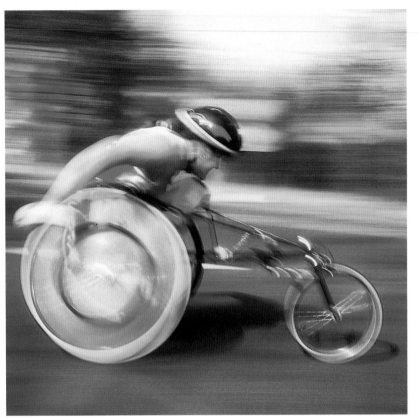

problem-orientated therapy, not a solution-orientated therapy. A problem shared can often be a problem doubled. Reliving a traumatic experience can often give a patient twice as much trauma to deal with. One of the reasons that counseling is not included in this guide is because many Western counselors are problem-orientated rather than solution-orientated. This is why people can be in therapy for many years. However, solution-orientated counseling, especially if it uses flower remedies or kinesiology release techniques can be very beneficial.

Embracing illness and "changing your mind"

If you try to fight an illness, you feed it energy that will make it stronger. The only way to beat an illness is to embrace it and learn from it. In this way you will be taking energy from your illness. The more you learn from an illness, the more energy you will take from it and the weaker it will become. This is another way in which you can "change your mind" and view illness from a new perspective. This power of changing your mind is available to every human being and the more you use it, the better you become at it. You can change your mind in the twinkling of an eye, which means the solution to any problem in your life is only a thought away.

Searching for solutions

There are some practitioners of mind therapies who are not helping people restore themselves to health. Any therapy that demands that you relive past traumas is a

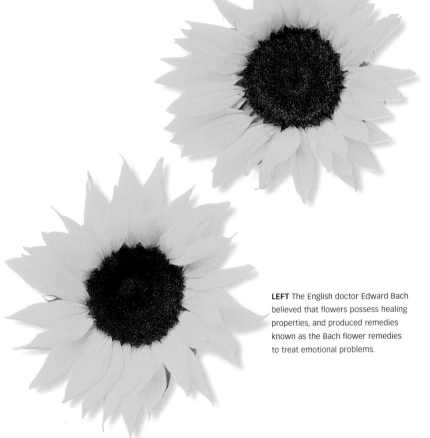

LEFT The English doctor Edward Bach believed that flowers possess healing properties, and produced remedies known as the Bach flower remedies to treat emotional problems.

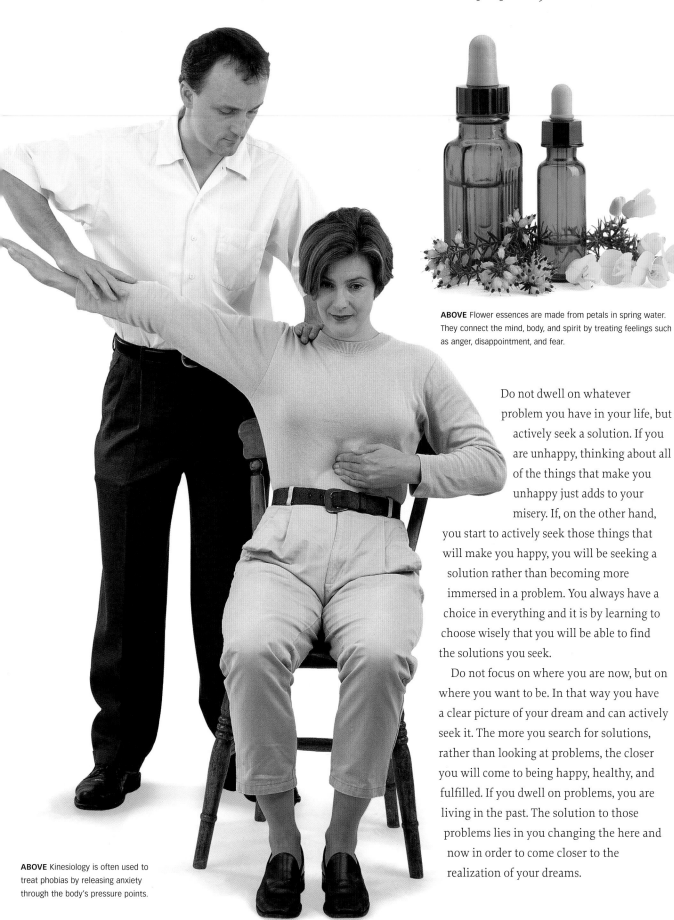

ABOVE Flower essences are made from petals in spring water. They connect the mind, body, and spirit by treating feelings such as anger, disappointment, and fear.

Do not dwell on whatever problem you have in your life, but actively seek a solution. If you are unhappy, thinking about all of the things that make you unhappy just adds to your misery. If, on the other hand, you start to actively seek those things that will make you happy, you will be seeking a solution rather than becoming more immersed in a problem. You always have a choice in everything and it is by learning to choose wisely that you will be able to find the solutions you seek.

Do not focus on where you are now, but on where you want to be. In that way you have a clear picture of your dream and can actively seek it. The more you search for solutions, rather than looking at problems, the closer you will come to being happy, healthy, and fulfilled. If you dwell on problems, you are living in the past. The solution to those problems lies in you changing the here and now in order to come closer to the realization of your dreams.

ABOVE Kinesiology is often used to treat phobias by releasing anxiety through the body's pressure points.

Visualization

The mind and body communicate in a language of metaphors. Dreams are often symbolic metaphors highlighting the solution to a problem or communicating something to us. The interpretation of dreams is the unlocking of these metaphors. Visualization is a way in which we can use the mind to communicate with the body and effect change using metaphors. The imagination creates a picture or scenario and then changes that scene to a healthier outcome. For instance, it has been shown that if a person with a broken bone visualizes the bone mending and re-growing, it speeds up the healing process.

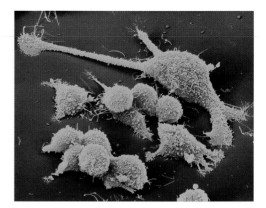

ABOVE Visualizing cancer cells being eaten or attacked by the cells of the immune system has been shown to complement conventional treatment and speed up recovery.

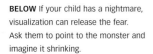

BELOW If your child has a nightmare, visualization can release the fear. Ask them to point to the monster and imagine it shrinking.

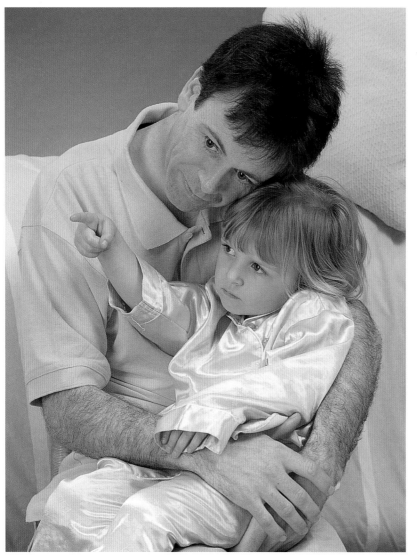

Visualization and children's nightmares

This technique can be used for adults or for children. If your child has a nightmare or bad dream you can use visualization with them to reenter that dream and change it. Ask them to point at any scary monsters with their index finger and tell them to imagine the monster shrinking down to a size that is no longer threatening. Now the tiny monster can be befriended and questioned about what it is coming to teach that child. If the dream has unpleasant things occurring, get the child to reimagine them and change the outcome to a happier one. Remember that there are no limits to the imagination. If the child is too big to fit into somewhere, they can shrink down to size and if they are too small, they can make themselves grow to giant proportions.

Psychoneuroimmunology

Psychoneuroimmunology is a new branch of Western medicine that is being used with great effect on cancer patients. As its name suggests, it involves using the mind to boost the immune system and fight disease. One of the reasons scientists think that the body's own immune system does not fight cancer is that cancer behaves in a unique way that fools the immune system. Whenever the body is invaded by an outside pathogen (i.e. a bacteria or virus), the pathogen attacks the cells of the body and kills them. When a cell dies, its cell membrane splits open and this alerts the immune system that something is wrong. Cancer, on the other hand, does not kill cells. Because cancer cell membranes remain intact, the immune system does not recognize that the body is under attack and therefore does not respond to the cancer.

Doctors have discovered that if a patient visualizes the cell membranes of the cancer cells within their body splitting, it seems to greatly improve the recovery and mortality rates of cancer patients. Cancer patients are also encouraged to visualize increased blood-cell production during chemotherapy and this again appears to be reducing side effects and speeding recovery.

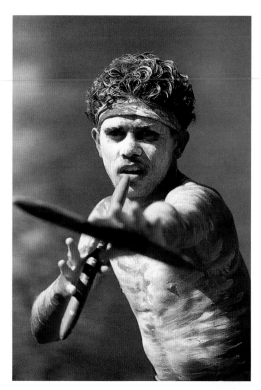

LEFT Aborigines use pointing sticks to draw out the demons they believe are causing sickness. Incantations are recited by a holy man while the patient is touched with the sticks.

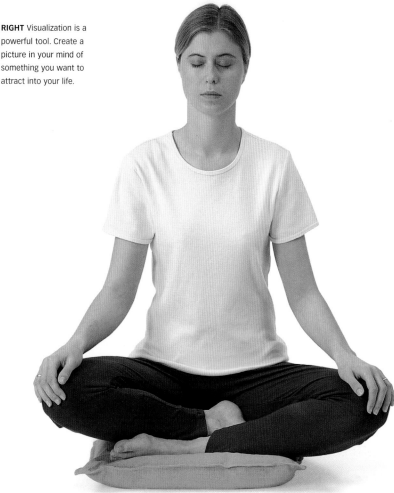

RIGHT Visualization is a powerful tool. Create a picture in your mind of something you want to attract into your life.

John and his recurring dream

Ten-year-old John kept having a recurring dream. Although the dream was not terribly frightening, it was troubling him enough that he did not want to go to bed at night. His mother sought the help of a complementary therapist who encouraged John to describe his dream. In the dream John was on his bed, but the bed was floating down a long corridor with doors on either side. John told the therapist that in the dream he felt a tremendous urge to go through the doors but he was frightened that if he left the safety of his bed, he might not be able to return. The therapist simply got John to relive his dream but to shrink the bed and himself down to a size where the bed would fit through the doors without him needing to leave it. This John did and having visualized looking through all the doors while safely on his bed, he never had the dream again. The therapist also taught John to always change his bad dreams to good ones if they troubled him and he was never fearful of sleep again.

Using visualization

The following visualization technique is for treating a headache but it can be used to treat any pain within the body. Find a warm, comfortable place to sit or lie down where you will not be disturbed for 5 minutes. Close your eyes and take a few slow, deep breaths to relax. Now focus your mind on the pain in your head. Try to imagine the shape of the pain (i.e. where exactly it is located) and give it a color. It may be a black blob or a red sphere for instance. When you have clearly pictured the pain's shape and color, imagine it as a liquid and mentally push it out through your third

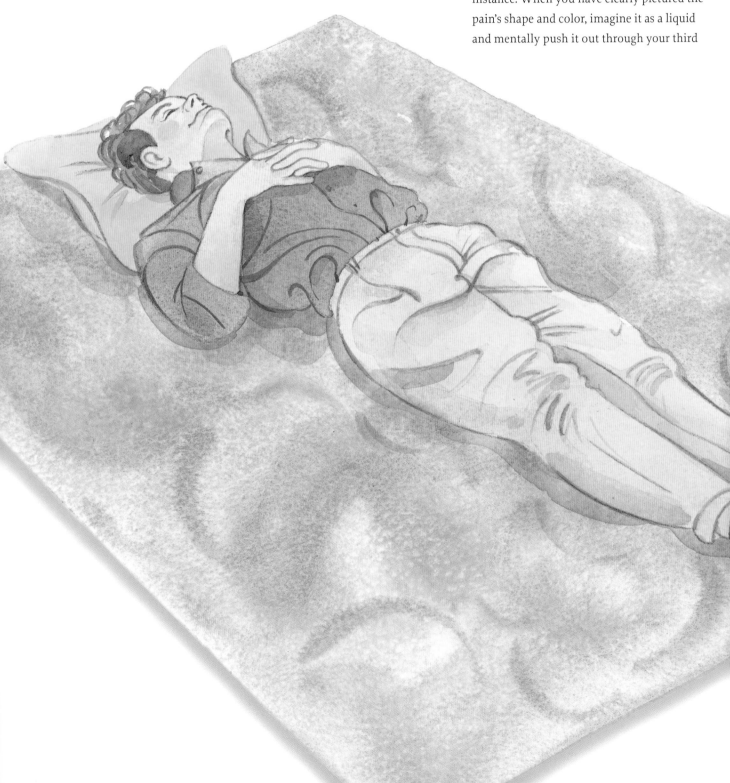

eye (on your forehead between your eyebrows) and into an imaginary glass. When you have done this, hold the glass up and see how full it is. Now imagine pouring that colored liquid down a drain and rinse the drain and glass out with water from an imaginary tap. Now check back inside your head and see if the shape and color of the pain has changed or if the pain has now gone. If the shape and color have changed, repeat the process of imagining the pain pouring out of your third eye and being rinsed away. This technique will resolve many headaches. For pain felt in other parts of the body, imagine the colored liquid rising up the spine, over the top of the head, and out through the third eye.

Visualization in everyday life

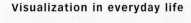

Whenever you experience any illness in any part of your body, from indigestion to major infections, imagine the affected part of the body healing itself, and it will speed up your journey back to health. For instance, if you have indigestion, you could visualize your stomach as a stormy sea becoming gradually more and more calm until it is completely serene. This will communicate to your body how you would like it to behave. At the same time, if you try to understand what your body is teaching you by noting any messages or images that spontaneously arise from your visualization, this too will speed up your recovery time. Do not underestimate the power of this technique. The more you use it, the more effective it will become and the more time you will be able to spend in happiness, health, and fulfillment.

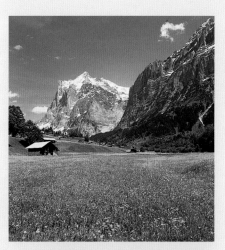

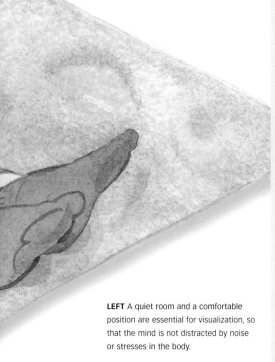

LEFT Prepare your mind to make a difficult decision by imagining a calm, serene mountain scene. If you see a human figure enter the scene, approach them and ask for their advice. This is your own wisdom speaking to you.

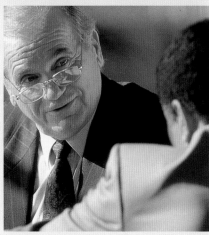

LEFT Before a job interview, visualize yourself answering questions with ease and watch the interviewer react with genuine interest. When you walk into the interview for real, your attitude will be calm and confident.

LEFT A quiet room and a comfortable position are essential for visualization, so that the mind is not distracted by noise or stresses in the body.

Meditation

Meditation is a technique that allows the body and mind to become calm and relaxed so as to facilitate spiritual enlightenment, self-realization, or healing. In simplest terms, it is sitting or lying down and relaxing. When the body and mind are in this state of tranquility, the body's energies run smoothly and more efficiently, allowing the body to heal itself and the mind to teach itself.

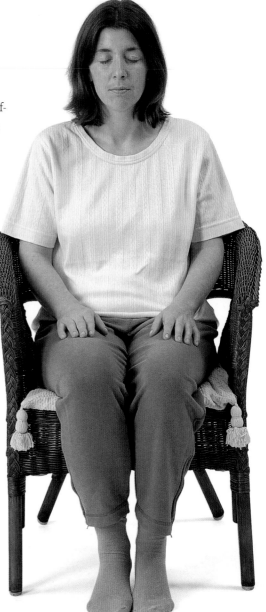

ABOVE Many people find sitting on a chair the most comfortable way to meditate. The chair should be firm with an upright back.

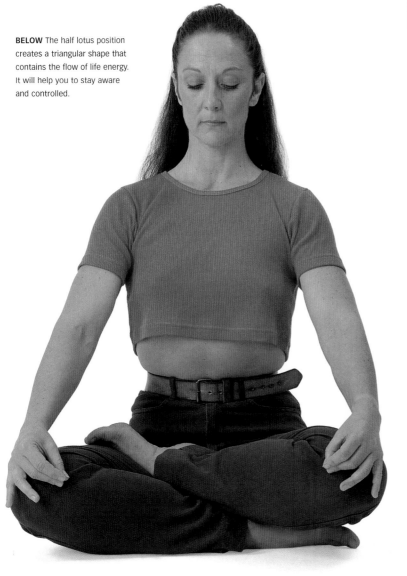

BELOW The half lotus position creates a triangular shape that contains the flow of life energy. It will help you to stay aware and controlled.

Meditation has been practiced in India and the Orient for thousands of years and it has now been established as a genuine help to the healing process. One of the most wonderful things about meditation is that it can be practiced by anyone at any age with no equipment at all and can be of great benefit to all who practice it. It simply requires a human being and time.

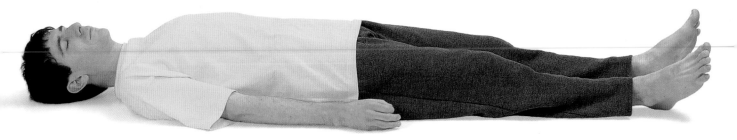

Postures for meditation

• Sitting on the floor: Sit against a wall with your back straight, your legs outstretched, and your feet together. Rest your hands lightly on your lap.

• Sitting on a chair: Sit on a firm, but comfortable chair with your feet together, flat on the floor. Again rest your hands lightly on your lap.

• Kneeling: Sit on your heels with your back straight and your head slightly inclined forward. Rest your hands on your lap.

• Lying down: Lie flat on your back with your legs flat or your knees bent with your feet flat on the floor. Rest your hands by your side.

• The lotus position: Sit with your legs crossed and with either one foot resting on the thigh of the other leg (the half lotus) or with both feet resting on the thighs (the full lotus). Place your hands in your lap or on your knees.

Breathing

During meditation all breathing should be done through the nose with the mouth closed. The breathing should be deep, slow, and relaxed.

Simple relaxation meditation

For this exercise you will need a comfortable, warm place to sit or lie where you will not be disturbed. If you have a telephone, unplug it or turn it off. Sit or lie in a comfortable position and relax. Close your eyes. Let all the worries and cares leave your mind and just concentrate on your breathing. Now, think of each part of your body relaxing. Begin at your toes and work up the body, mentally relaxing every muscle until your whole body is in a state of deep relaxation. Allow thoughts to wash over you and just concentrate on your breathing. If your mind becomes occupied, just refocus your energies and concentrate once more on your breathing. Once you have relaxed your whole body, you can enjoy this meditative state for 15–30 minutes as time allows. It usually takes at least 20 minutes for a novice to achieve a meditative state.

When you feel the time to end the meditation has come, gently take a few deep breaths and open your eyes. You should rise slowly to avoid serious physical exertion immediately after meditating. Give your mind and body time to acclimatize before doing anything mentally or physically strenuous. If you feel a bit "spacey" after meditating, try walking barefoot on grass or doing a simple chi kung exercise to help ground your energy.

ABOVE Only meditate lying down if you are feeling alert. If you are tired, you may fall asleep.

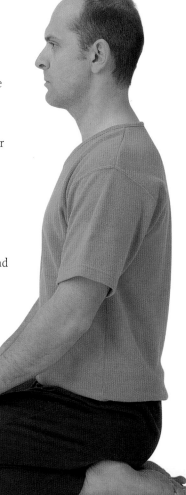

RIGHT Kneeling will help you to stay relaxed but attentive. At the end of the meditation, rub your legs before standing to help prevent unsteadyness.

Learning meditation

There are many clubs and courses teaching meditation. Many family doctors now refer their patients to meditation teachers and some hold regular meditation groups in their clinics since it has been shown to help combat any form of stress. Meditation is also often taught in yoga, tai chi, and chi kung classes. Indeed tai chi is often described as "moving meditation." There are many good books teaching simple meditation, as well as tapes that give guided meditations. Meditation is very easy to learn and the more you use it, the more powerful it becomes.

LEFT In yoga, the body is the instrument of the mind. As the mind becomes less resistant, the body stretches further and the asanas (postures) become easier.

Guided meditation

Guided meditation is a form of meditation where the person meditating is directed or guided on what to do and how to use their imagination. It can bring about deep states of relaxation and inner calm. The guided meditation on the right is designed to be read aloud. You can either get a friend to read it to you or you can tape it and play it back to yourself.

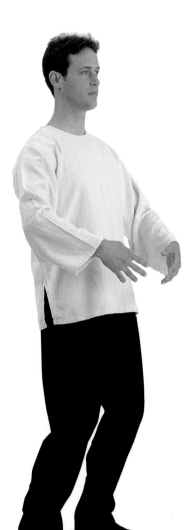

ABOVE In chi kung, controlling the breath brings peace and regulates the internal organs.

RIGHT Practiced in a meditative way, tai chi steps draw energy toward the body through the palms of the hands and soles of the feet.

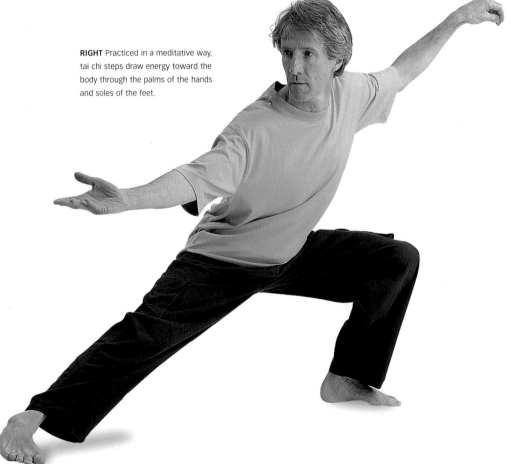

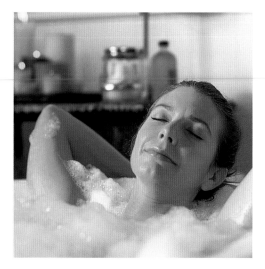

ABOVE Guided meditation can take you to an imaginary place of absolute relaxation. You can return to the same place whenever you find a quiet moment.

First find a quiet place where you will not be disturbed and sit or lie in a meditative posture. Quieten your mind and listen to the words being spoken. Let your imagination take you on a journey to find a special place. You can create any natural scene that makes you feel calm and relaxed, and experience its colors, scents, and sounds.

Once you have mastered traveling to your special place, you can do it anytime without the guide. You can travel there in the bathtub, on a train, in the park, anywhere. All you need to do is close your eyes and imagine. Many people find traveling to their special place a very good stressbuster. If you do try it, it is worth remembering to give yourself time to return gently to normal consciousness when you leave your special place. Next time you are faced with a problem and cannot find a solution, take 10 minutes to go to your special place and relax. The peace and space experienced by your subconscious mind will give you the opportunity to work on the problem while you relax. You may well find that after you have meditated, the solution pops into your conscious mind.

> **❝** *Relax your mind . . . relax your breathing . . . just observe the slow movement of your breathing . . in . . and out . . . feel your body becoming more and more relaxed . . . now allow your mind to drift . . . to drift to a beautiful, natural place . . . it is a peaceful place full of wonderful plants and flowers . . . this is a place of complete safety where nothing can harm you... take a few moments to look around and enjoy nature's beauty . . . this is your special place . . . it is a place where nothing and no one can harm you . . . it is a place of stillness . . . and calm . . . In order to help you fix this place in your imagination . . . notice the light. . . what time of day is it? . . . Notice the temperature . . . is it warm or cool? . . . Now look around and take note of any plants, flowers and animals that you see . . . This special place is a place of calm and freedom so explore it, secure in the knowledge that you are safe . . . if you allow your mind to drift with the breeze you will find yourself flying or floating gently around this place . . . Listen to the sounds and follow them if you want to . . . . . just enjoy all that you are experiencing . . . and know that this is a place where you can truly relax.* **❞**

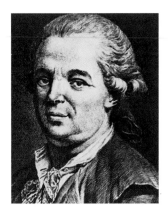

ABOVE Franz Mesmer believed that magnets moved an invisible healing fluid around the body.

Hypnosis

The word hypnosis originates from the Greek word hypnos meaning, "sleep." For centuries medicine men and shamans throughout the world have used hypnotic states to treat mental and physical illnesses. In modern times, the work of an Austrian doctor, Franz Anton Mesmer (1734–1815), brought hypnosis into the public eye. Mesmer claimed to be able to cure illnesses through his "animal magnetism" and he did this by creating a type of trance in his patients (they were "mesmerized"). A few years later a surgeon called James Esdaile (1808–1859) was working in Calcutta using only hypnosis as anesthetic. When modern anesthetics were discovered, hypnosis fell out of favor but it is now enjoying a great revival. Hypnotherapy, as it is now called, is generally regarded as a very real and potentially powerful healing tool.

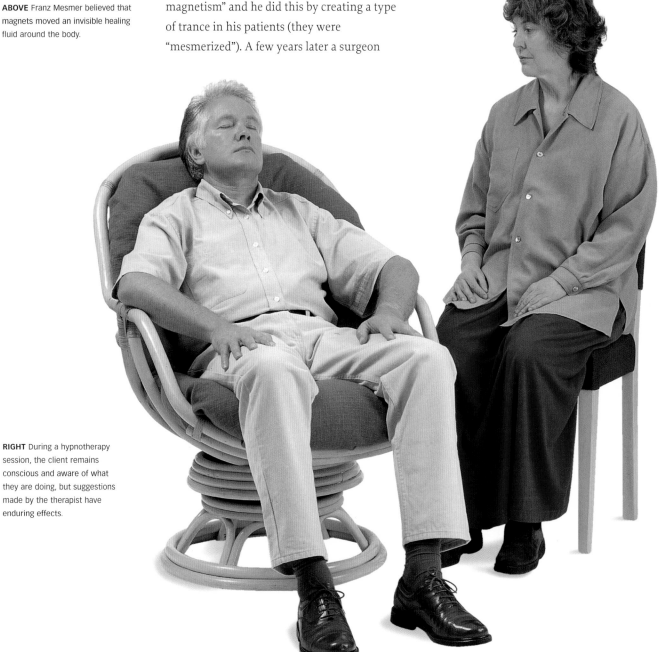

RIGHT During a hypnotherapy session, the client remains conscious and aware of what they are doing, but suggestions made by the therapist have enduring effects.

Who benefits from hypnotherapy?

Hypnotherapy has been successfully used to treat a range of illnesses including irritable bowel syndrome, migraines, headaches, skin disorders, asthma, and depression. It has also been used for pain relief during childbirth and dental surgery. Perhaps the best known use of hypnotherapy is in the treatment of fears and phobias, but it is also used to improve self-confidence, reduce stress, and treat addictions.

Finding a therapist

In many countries there are no rules governing hypnotherapy and hypnotherapists can practice with little or no qualifications. It is important when looking for a therapist to make sure they have been properly trained. Ask them what experience they have in treating your particular problem. Most importantly though, you must feel comfortable with the energy of the therapist. They will be delving into your subconscious, so it is important that you are able to trust them.

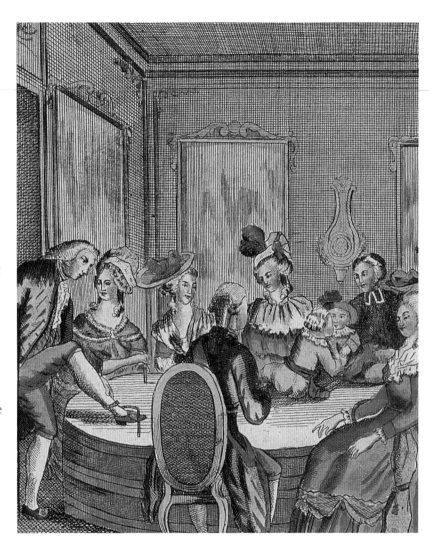

RIGHT Mesmer moved to Paris in 1778, where theatrical demonstrations of "animal magnetism" soon became popular.

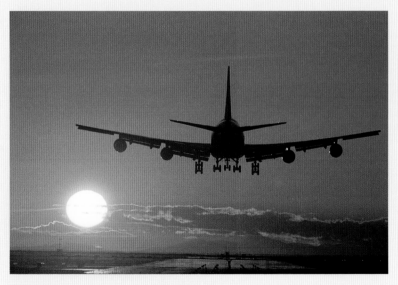

Overcoming a fear of flying

Alan was a successful businessman with a phobia of flying. This was not a problem for him until his business had the opportunity to expand abroad, and the only thing stopping Alan was his fear of flying. He consulted a hypnotherapist to try to solve the problem.

In his first session, the therapist hypnotized Alan and got him to imagine looking at a plane in a hanger and walking on it. The second session involved Alan imagining boarding a plane, sitting down in a relaxed state while it taxied up and down the runway, and then leaving the plane. In the third session the plane took off on a short flight and by the fifth session Alan was imagining taking long flights over Europe and North America.

Shortly after his sixth session, Alan flew from England to the United States and back again on his first ever transatlantic business trip; he has never experienced any problems with flying since.

Neurolinguistic programming

Neurolinguistic programming, known as NLP, is a simple, yet very powerful technique for unlocking the mind and effecting positive change within an individual. This technique studies how humans think and experience the world, and creates mental models of these patterns. Using these mental models, quick and efficient techniques for changing self-limiting or negative thoughts and behaviors have been developed.

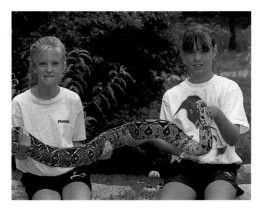

ABOVE Neurolinguistic progamming can banish phobias by changing the patient's outlook and reactions. It can remove the fear from situations that the patient finds difficult.

NLP has many different techniques but they all work in a similar manner. The following is an example for treating a snake phobia.

If you ask a person with a phobia of snakes to picture one, they would almost certainly create an image in their minds of a snake that is completely oversized and very close to their body. In reality, snakes are rarely threatening in size and are very likely to be far more frightened of you than you should be of them. But try telling that to someone with a phobia of snakes!

An NLP practitioner would ask the question,

"If another person can have fun playing with their pet snake, what can we learn about them that we could teach the phobic person so that they can play with snakes too?"

The snakelover would most likely have an image of snakes that was proportionally correct and at a reasonable distance from the body. Recognizing this difference, the NLP practitioner uses one of many techniques to help the phobic person relearn their reaction

ABOVE The phobic sees a snake as a large, threatening animal. NLP can adjust this image, making it more realistic.

to snakes so that it more like the reaction of
the snakelover. Although this may sound
complicated, in reality a competent NLP
practitioner can often successfully treat
phobias in a single 30-minute session.

What can NLP help?

Perhaps a better question is what can NLP not
help? This is because NLP is an approach to
health and healing that relies on flexibility.
If what you are doing is not working, NLP
teaches that it is only by initiating change that
a solution will be found. NLP offers pathways
and attitudes to change that can be applied to
any problem or illness.

There are many courses teaching NLP and
one of the best ways to experience it is to learn
how to do it. There are a growing number of
competent practitioners and most are members
of accredited organizations with a code of ethics
that can be viewed by anyone. The best way to
judge a practitioner is through questioning
their experience and perceiving their energy
(i.e. do you feel comfortable with them?).

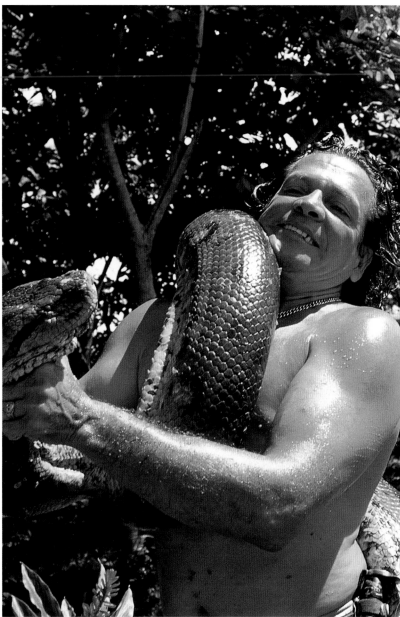

ABOVE In countries where snakes are part of the natural habitat,
instinctual fear of the animal is far less prevalent.

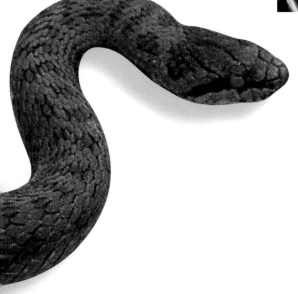

NLP presuppositions

NLP is based on a series of presuppositions that support the attitude that initiating change is the only way to find solutions. Practitioners of NLP usually have their own set of presuppositions but the following are the most common:

• Communication is more than what you are saying – the body communicates constantly in many nonverbal ways that can be "read" i.e. body posture.

• People already have all the resources they need to effect change – the resources just weren't in the right place at the right time.

• Choice is better than no choice – movement is better than stagnation.

• There is no such thing as failure, only feedback – every response is useful because it

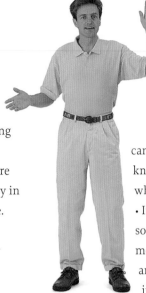

LEFT If you are anticipating a difficult situation, either at work or at home, visualize yourself responding positively to the situation in your mind beforehand.

can be a valuable source of knowledge and insight when viewed objectively.

• If someone can do something, then it can be modeled and taught to anyone else – that includes you.

• The map is not the territory – we cannot take in and remember every piece of information that comes to us in the world, so we create a "map of the territory" and then refer to the map for information that helps us to navigate the world we live in. By teaching a person to change their map, we can change their reality.

• The meaning of your communication is the response you get – if the way you communicate with another person is met with a response of anger, try communicating in a different way.

• If you aren't getting the response you want, try something different – see previous presupposition.

• People work perfectly – there is no such thing as a dysfunctional person. Every person is functioning perfectly in what they are doing even if it is ruining their life i.e. when people do self-destructive things, they do them very well! Find out how a person is functioning now and you can show them how they can change that function into something they consider more desirable.

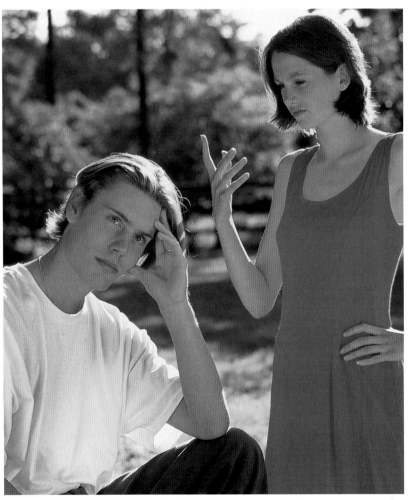

LEFT Be aware of how your posture and movements affect other people. Lack of eye contact and shielding the face can make a difficult situation worse.

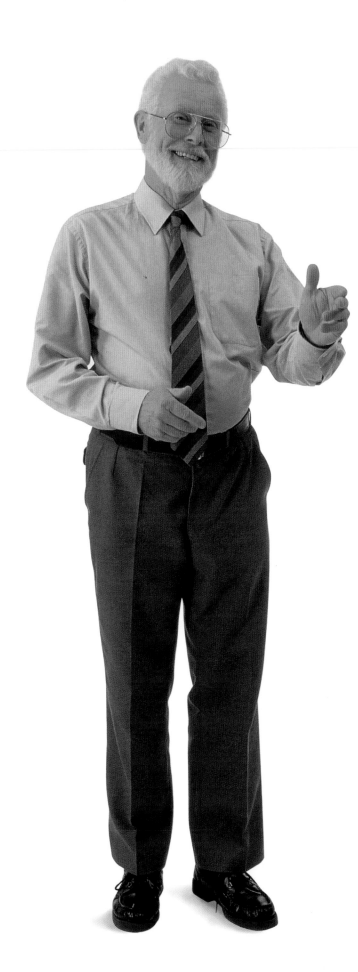

Viewing a situation

In order to change how you view a situation using NLP techniques, you will need a few minutes in a quiet place, the directions that follow and your brain!

Think of a time when you were having an unpleasant conflict with someone else. This could be your partner, a child, a work colleague, or anyone. Reexperience this situation in your mind, noticing the other person's reactions, their physical postures, their gestures etc.

Clear this image from your mind and now reexperience the situation as the other person. Using the information you have just gathered about the other person, step into their shoes and, as you progress through the experience, imagine what your feelings and attitudes are as that other person. Note the new information you gain from this new perspective.

Clear this image from your mind and now experience the situation from an outsider's point of view. Watch the experience unfold from a neutral space and note any new information gained by this new perspective.

You now have three different ways of perceiving the situation. With all this new knowledge, you should be able to view the overall situation with much greater objectivity and you should be able to understand and empathize with the other person more efficiently. This will enable you to not take their behavior personally.

Radionics

Radionics is a method of healing at a distance. It does not require the patient's presence for diagnosis or treatment. It uses specially designed instruments in conjunction with radiesthesia (medical dowsing). Radionics is a science concerned with the energy patterns that are emitted from all forms of matter. In radionic therapy, any imbalances or distortions in a patient's energy patterns can be diagnosed and measured so that a trained practitioner can build up a blueprint of the patient which incorporates their physical, emotional, and spiritual levels. Treatment is designed to restore the patient's energy pattern to a harmonious resonance that then allows the body's own healing energies to complete the cure.

Dr. Albert Abrams (1863–1924) first discovered the principles of radionics while working in the United States as a leading specialist in diseases of the nervous system. A chance discovery made during the routine examination of a patient led him to revolutionize his whole approach to medicine, going way beyond the boundaries of the accepted medical and scientific thought at that time. He soon devised a new method of diagnosis through reading the energy patterns of different diseases, and later designed instruments to correct the imbalances these diseases caused in his patients. The actual term "radiesthesia" was coined by Abbé Mermet, a Swiss priest who applied the ancient art of dowsing to medicine in the 1920s. Modern radionics is a synthesis of medical dowsing combined with the diagnostic model created by Dr. Abrams.

Radionic treatment today

When a patient applies to a practitioner, they are sent a detailed diagnostic form to fill in. This is completed and returned to the practitioner along with a sample of the patient's hair or blood (called "a witness"). The "witness" is used so that the practitioner can connect with the patient's unique genetic blueprint held within the sample. The

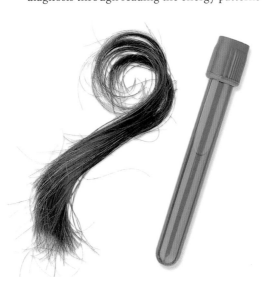

LEFT Samples of the patient's hair and blood emit energy patterns which a radionics practitioner measures and uses to make a diagnosis. Corrective energy can be sent to the patient via the samples.

practitioner then carries out his diagnosis and sends treatment(s) to the patient to remedy the disharmonies and imbalances he has diagnosed. These treatments are sent via radionic instruments to the patient and it does not matter whether the patient is in the same room as the practitioner or on the other side of the world. The "energies" sent to the patient may be the energy patterns of organs, minerals, vitamins, homeopathic remedies, herbs, or antidote patterns to a particular bacteria, virus, or other pathogen.

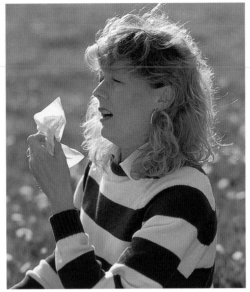

LEFT Hay fever and asthma often respond to radionic treatment. The technique has also been used to treat digestive problems, musculoskeletal discomfort, and stress.

Who benefits from radionics?

It should be said that not all patients respond to radionic treatment, but those that do can show remarkable results. Radionics has helped people with long-standing diseases such as asthma, allergies, hypertension, mental illness, and stress. To a radionic practitioner, a patient's named disease or symptoms are seen merely as manifestations of much deeper, underlying imbalances. The practitioner seeks to treat these imbalances, which then allows the body to fight the disease itself.

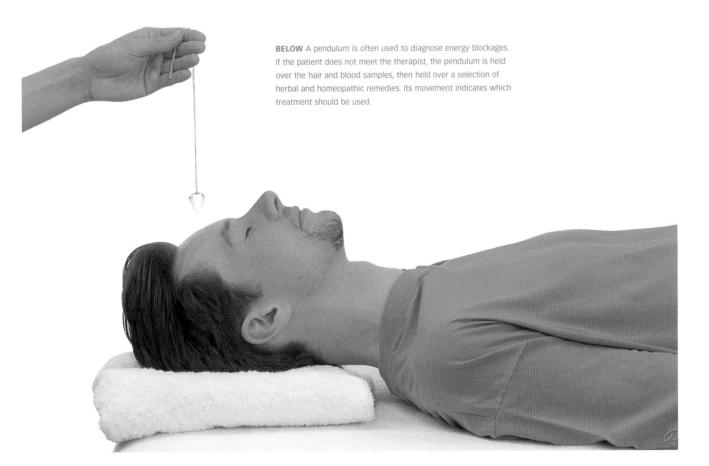

BELOW A pendulum is often used to diagnose energy blockages. If the patient does not meet the therapist, the pendulum is held over the hair and blood samples, then held over a selection of herbal and homeopathic remedies. Its movement indicates which treatment should be used.

Esoteric healing

The word esoteric means "Designed for, or appropriate to, an inner circle of disciples; communicated to, or intelligible to, the initiated only." It implies something that is hidden from general understanding and this is true of all of the therapies in this section. The people who practice these therapies were invariably taught on a one to one basis. There are many books that discuss esoteric healing therapies but learning them is achieved through personal communication. Each of the therapies relies on faith rather than science, although scientific proof of their power is beginning to arise.

The practice of any type of esoteric healing requires a special knowledge of energy and of how energy works that goes beyond the dimensions of space and time. The following teachings about energy are true, but at present unprovable by science. This does not mean that they should be ignored.

Energy and the universe

• Everything that you come into contact with is energy and running throughout all of creation is the divine spark of life. People have many names for the source of this spark: God, Buddha, Allah, Jehovah, Shiva, Osiris, and the Universe to name but a few.

• Every thought you have is an energy form that goes out into the universe. The energy you express in thought and deed is the energy you get back. It is the law of karma that "as you sow, so shall you reap."

• For anything to be healthy, it must be devoid of negative emotions and filled only with love. This love can be transferred to anything to make it more balanced and harmonious, whether it is another human being, an animal, a plant, or a crystal. All esoteric healing comes from a perspective of love.

• Through mastery of the ego, the body can become a channel for divine, healing love that can be transferred to another human being through the power of thought, prayer, or touch.

• The universe is a multi-dimensional, multilayered thing and energies can travel across these dimensions when the correct intent is applied to them.

• All human energy is directed and moved by the human mind.

RIGHT Gautama Buddha, "the enlightened one," abandoned his earthly ambitions to lead a life of contemplation.

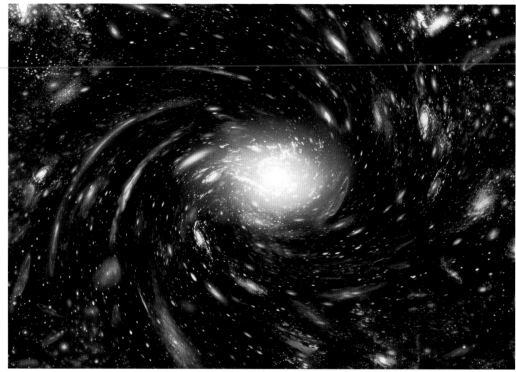

LEFT Every action creates a reaction, since energy can travel through every dimension of the universe. Periods of meditation open the mind to endless possibilities.

• Whenever you think about another person, some part of their being registers and acknowledges that thought.

• The web of life connects everything in creation. If you hurt another person, you are only hurting yourself. If you heal another person, you are healing yourself. Every positive change you make in your life has a positive effect on everyone you meet from the moment you make that change through eternity.

Many of these concepts are so alien to us that we dismiss them and esoteric healing remains on the fringes of society. This is sad because if we open our minds to the limitless possibilities of the universe, we will find that these therapies are totally consistent with the science of creation. The science of creation is the true and accurate science of the workings of the universe. It is beyond the human mind to fully understand and a far cry from the science of man, which is really no more than a set of theories that best fit the facts as we choose to see them!

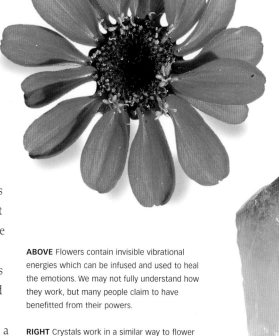

ABOVE Flowers contain invisible vibrational energies which can be infused and used to heal the emotions. We may not fully understand how they work, but many people claim to have benefitted from their powers.

RIGHT Crystals work in a similar way to flower essences – their vibrational energies can pass directly into the body through its aura or into water to make healing essences.

Spiritual healing

Spiritual healing has nothing to do with spiritualism. Spiritualism refers to a religion and is comparable with any of the world's religions. Spiritual healing is a nonreligious therapy that acknowledges the fact that we are spiritual beings living in a spiritual universe. A dictionary definition of the word "spiritual" defines it as: "Of spirit, as opposed to matter; of the soul, especially as acted on by God; of, proceeding from, God; holy, divine, inspired." So when the word "spiritual" is attached to the word "healing" it defines a type of therapy that acknowledges a divine source. It acknowledges that healing comes from God, however you may perceive him, her, or it.

All spiritual healers acknowledge that they are channels of spiritual energies that flow from the divine. If a person calling themselves a "spiritual healer" denies that fact, they are not only denying the source of healing, they are denying God and denying the existence of those inhabitants of the spiritual realms that guide and help to heal humans on their life-paths.

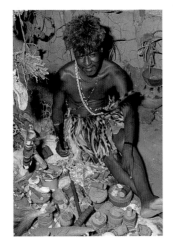

ABOVE Witch doctors go into a trance to seek guidance from the spirit world, and have been revered by tribal societies throughout history.

BELOW Spiritual healers tune in to the patient's aura to awaken the healing process. They often detect energy imbalances by using sweeping movements to find hot or cold areas, then hold their hands above these areas and channel divine energy toward them.

Spiritual healing and cancer

Recent studies have shown that spiritual healing appears to help recovery from major illnesses and especially cancer. Patients who had spiritual healing as well as chemotherapy reported fewer side effects and appeared to recover more quickly.

Finding a spiritual healer

All major churches and religions have their own spiritual healers. They may come under the title of healer, priest, shaman, medicine-man, or pastor but they all practice the same therapy. There are also nondenominational and nonreligious organizations that offer spiritual healing. In most cases this therapy is given for no charge or for the exchange of a gift or donation rather than for a set fee. Anyone charging large amounts of money for "spiritual healing" is not healing from a spiritual perspective, but from a worldly one. Avoid these people at all costs!

The healing power of prayer

All spiritual paths acknowledge the healing power of prayer. You do not have to be religious to pray. Some would say that you don't even have to believe in God. Prayer is a positive thought-form sent out into the universe. If it is a pure thought-form bathed in unconditional and unselfish love, devoid of emotions such as greed or envy, it will have a positive effect. The best prayers are ones devoid of preconceived ideas and conditions. Rather than praying for a new car, pray for a solution to your transportation problems.

Rather than praying for specific healing, pray that the sick person might find peace within themselves and learn the lessons that life is trying to teach them. This type of prayer is more likely to receive a positive answer.

On the other hand, stories are told about people who have seen miracles and specific healing take place through persistent and conscientious prayer. Through sending positive, loving prayers over a period of time, perhaps an accumulative effect takes place that initiates change. Certainly it is a form of spiritual healing that we can all perform and that deserves exploration.

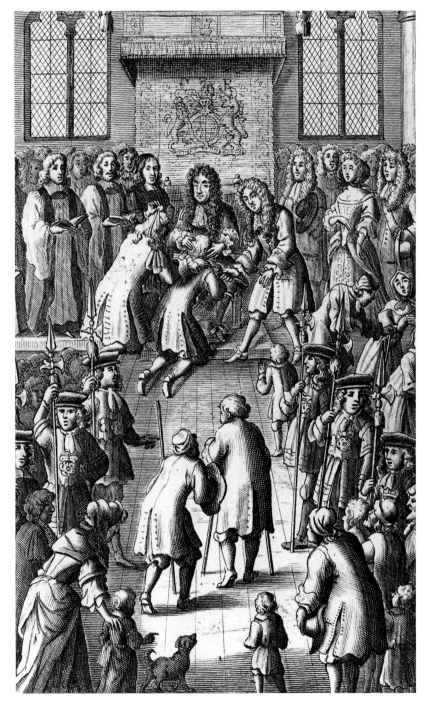

BELOW In medieval times, the plague was thought to be God's punishment for man's sins. The royal hands of Charles II of England, said to have healing properties, touched many sufferers.

Remote healing

Remote or absent healing is a form of spiritual healing that does not require the healer and patient to be in the same place. They can be in separate places anywhere in the world. Practitioners use meditation, prayer, and visualization to form a divine or mystical link to the patient that is not bound by distance. The healer then sends channeled healing energies to the patient, activating the patient's own inner healing abilities.

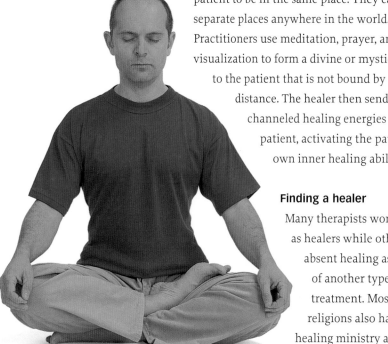

ABOVE During a meditation session, energy can cross huge distances to create an intuitive link between a healer and their patient. The half-lotus pose helps to concentrate the energy.

Finding a healer

Many therapists work only as healers while others use absent healing as part of another type of treatment. Most religions also have a healing ministry and an approach can often be made through a minister, priest, or other religious worker. In Britain, the General Medical Council allows a family doctor to refer a patient to a healer, provided that the doctor remains in overall charge of the patient's treatment and health. There are even family doctors that now provide absent healing alongside their orthodox treatments.

Most healers do not diagnose patients nor do they require a diagnosis to treat them. Healing is usually performed as a support to other therapies (orthodox or alternative), not as a replacement for them. Many absent healers ask their patients to sit or lie and meditate at a prearranged time when they will send the patient healing. Others ask nothing of their patients except a name. All absent healing should be free of charge.

How to send healing

Method one

Set aside a time when you will not be disturbed. Lie or sit in a meditative posture and relax your body and mind. Visualize the person you want to send healing to. Imagine them being bathed in beautiful white light until every part of their being is shining. Send loving and healing thoughts to them, visualizing the energy of those thoughts as pure white light washing them clean of all illness and imbalance. When you feel ready, slowly bring your attention back into the room while holding a picture of the person in your mind looking and feeling happy, healthy, and fulfilled. Finally release that image from your mind and rinse your hands and face in cool water to refresh your energy.

RIGHT The patient receives the absent healer's energy, which flows into the body and encourages self-healing. Complete faith in the process will make it more effective.

Method two

On a piece of paper, write a simple healing prayer such as: "I ask that ——— may find peace and balance in their lives and feel the loving healing energies of God (or the universe)."

Read the prayer aloud and then fold the piece of paper so that the prayer is hidden. Light a candle and place the piece of paper under the candlestick. As the candle burns, your healing thoughts will be continually traveling to that person. Alternatively, you may light the piece of paper with the candle and let it burn while visualizing your prayer traveling to the person and activating their own healing energies.

These simple actions can have profound effects. Have faith in these techniques and believe that anything is possible.

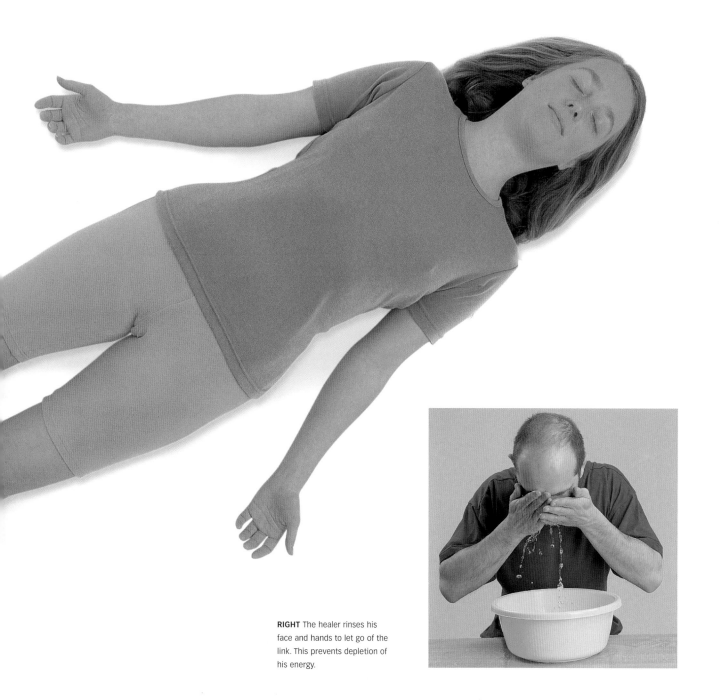

RIGHT The healer rinses his face and hands to let go of the link. This prevents depletion of his energy.

Shamanic healing

The word shaman originally referred to a Siberian priest-doctor but is now used to describe any medicine person from an Earth-based spiritual belief system be it Celtic, Native American, African, or from elsewhere.

All shamans share a common belief that the physical world is just one of many planes in a multi-dimensional universe. All shamans understand energy and energy healing and incorporate it into their shamanic healing practices.

LEFT Native American shamans assume a new identity by wearing symbolic masks during their ceremonial rites. Demonic disguises enable them to pass unnoticed in the spirit world.

Shamanic essences

Shamanic essences are energy medicines, which are used primarily for connecting us to a greater reality. By utilizing the shamanic qualities of the elements, and of plants, trees, animals, planets, moon, and stars, essences are produced that work completely in harmony with the natural world. They each have unique healing and balancing abilities and mankind, as a member of the animal kingdom, can connect to his brothers and sisters in the natural world in a deeply profound, spiritual way. The animals become our guides and teachers, and can show us how to walk the path of the heart and so live at peace with others and ourselves. No animal is harmed during the making of these essences, they openly choose to cooperate while the essence is in production, in order to help their human brothers and sisters realize their relationship to the other kingdoms on this earth. Animal essences are created in a similar way to flower and gem essences. Each essence contains the vibrational energy of the individual animal and all its attributes; for example, owl for clarity. For this reason alone, these energy medicines have an important role to play in guiding mankind back to a more enlightened and harmonious way of life.

The San Pedro cactus contains the hallucinogenic drug mescaline.

BELOW Worshipers in Salvador, Brazil, smoke powerful herbs in a Candomble ceremony, inducing a state of trance which allows the dancers to be possessed by the gods.

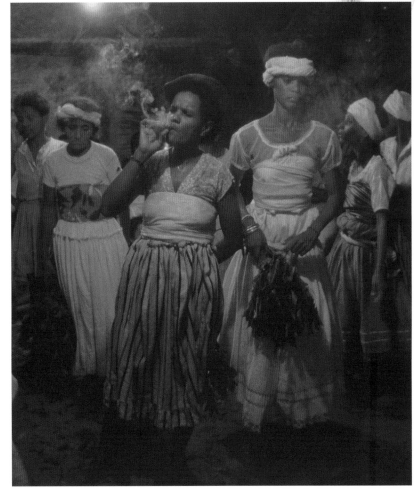

Smudging

Smudging or "sweeping the smoke" is a Native American purification ceremony used for healing and before the performance of sacred rituals. Similar practices can be found throughout the world, including the burning of incense in the Catholic Church. The Native Americans use local herbs such as sage or sweetgrass while other cultures use powerful resins such as frankincense.

Roll some sage or a similar herb in your hands imparting into it any prayers, wishes, or positive thoughts that feel appropriate. Light the herb until it is smoking well and then place it in a container or pot so that it does not burn you. Using a feather, fan, or your hand, waft the smoke around the head, allowing the patient to breath in the smoke. Then, beginning at the feet, waft the smoke all around the front of the body working your way up toward the head. When you reach

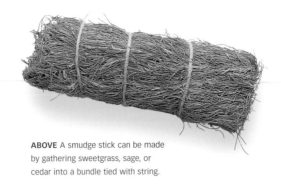

ABOVE A smudge stick can be made by gathering sweetgrass, sage, or cedar into a bundle tied with string.

the head, flick the feather, fan or your hand to remove any negative energy that the smoke may have picked up from the person's aura. Work your way down the back toward the feet. Get the patient to lift up each foot and smudge underneath it. This will help to connect their energies to the earth. Repeat this, circling around the patient in a clockwise direction. When done, offer a prayer of thanks and give your patient a hug.

RIGHT Smudging beneath the feet has the effect of grounding the patient or giving them roots. Smudging around the body purifies the aura. While you smudge, waft the smoke around the patient with a feather, a fan, or your hand.

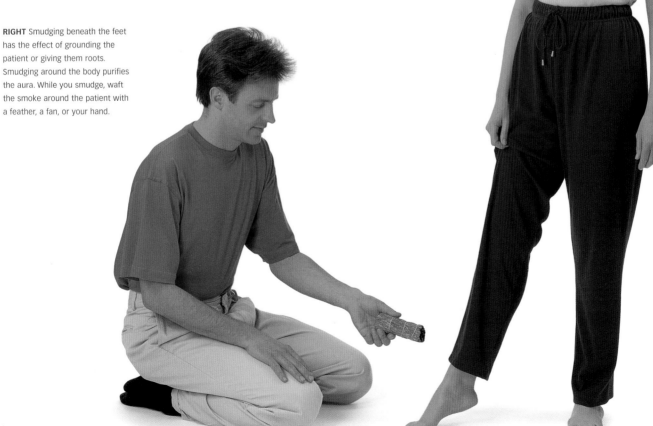

The sacred sweatlodge is a Celtic and Native American purification ceremony that some call a spiritual sauna. It is a powerful and profound healing ritual that can initiate great change in the individuals taking part. A person's first visit to a sweatlodge is often a life-changing experience.

Stones that have been heated on a fire are brought into a covered bender (hazel or willow dwelling) or lodge and placed in a central pit. The lodge represents the womb of Mother Earth and the fire represents the divine spark of the creator. The lodge is closed and herbs and prayers are offered up. Then water is poured onto the hot rocks creating steam that opens all the pores of the body allowing toxins to be released. Sweatlodges can get very hot and anyone with a debilitating illness or heart problems should not undertake this type of therapy without seeking medical advice.

The following is one person's description of their first sweatlodge experience:
"It was a cool, crisp evening as 16 of us gathered around the fire wearing nothing but shorts or sarongs. The stones had been heating for 2 hours and after each being smudged, we entered the lodge. As we entered we each called out "mitakuye oyasin," which is Lakota for "we are all related" to affirm our connection to creation. Seven red-hot stones were brought into the lodge and placed in the middle. The door was closed and all was black except for the dull glow of the rocks. After singing a song and saying some prayers, the one who was pouring the water liberally doused the stones. The steam rose and it suddenly became very hot. People called on animal and plant spirits or energies to come into the lodge and help with the healing. Prayers and songs were interspersed with jokes and laughter that banished any feelings of fear or discomfort. After a while the water-pourer

called out the words "mitakuye oyasin" and the fire-keeper opened the door letting in the cold night air.

The second round began with seven more stones being brought into the lodge. This time healing herbs were placed on the hot stones so that the lodge was filled with fragrant scents. This was the healing round and healing prayers and songs accompanied the sound of

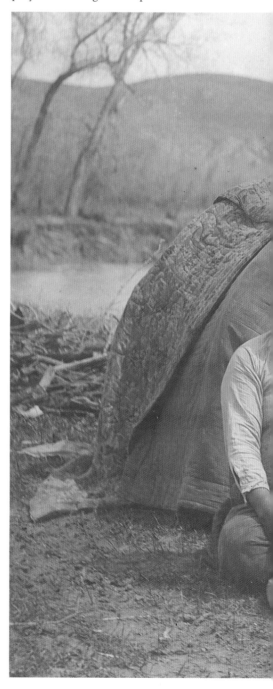

hissing steam as more water was poured on the rocks. After a while the call to open the door was given and we all breathed in the cool fresh air once more. The third round was the prayer round. Seven more stones were brought into the lodge and we each took a turn at saying a simple prayer. At the end of each prayer more water was put on the rocks. The heat became almost unbearable and I was glad when the door was finally opened. The final seven stones were brought into the lodge for the fourth and last round. Prayers of thanks were offered up to the creator and to all the good spirits for our experiences and learning during the sweatlodge. The last of the water was poured on the stones and shortly after the door was opened. We all walked into the clear night feeling invigorated and renewed."

BELOW Native Americans in Crow Village, Montana, pause in the preparation of a sweatlodge shaped like a pregnant belly for a purifying rite of passage.

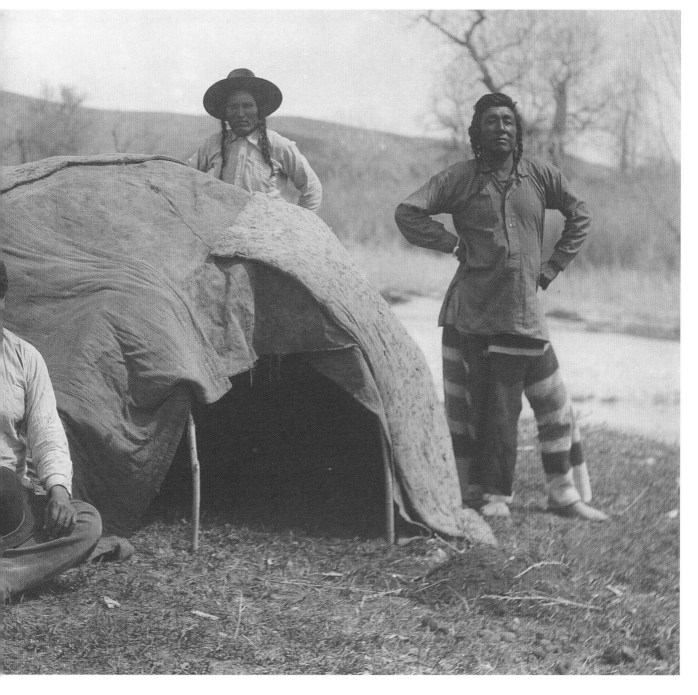

Crystals and gems

Crystals and gems have been in existence for hundreds of thousands of years as part of the structure of the living Earth. Their natural beauty has been prized by many ancient civilizations and their individual qualities have been utilized not only for decoration, but also for ceremonies, healing, and divination. One of the earliest records of crystals having healing properties comes from 1500 B.C.E. A piece of papyrus dating from that time called the "Papyrus Ebers" gives very detailed and specific knowledge about the individual healing properties of many crystals.

Crystals are composed of naturally occurring minerals and have a very ordered structure. The size of a crystal can vary from microscopic to bigger than you are! Many crystals are formed from molten lava rising from the Earth's core. Some are formed through minerals being dissolved and then deposited by water, while others are deposited by escaping gases coming up through the Earth's crust. Crystals, because of their regular structure, can carry and amplify healing energies. Our own bodies contain many crystalline structures within them and this means that we resonate very closely to the energies of crystals.

Using crystals in energy healing

Crystals are used in a variety of ways for energy healing. They may be held, worn, placed on an area of pain or sickness, or used to energize water, which is then drunk by the patient. There are therapists who specialize in crystal healing, although anyone can benefit from working on themselves with crystals without any formal training. Colored crystals have healing properties relating to their color (see Color healing, page 180) and each type of crystal has its own unique healing properties.

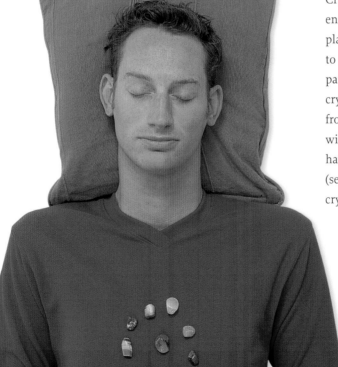

LEFT Crystals placed around the heart chakra encourage feelings of love and compassion and create a sense of unity with all living things.

Cleansing a crystal

If you are planning to purchase some crystals to use on yourself, it is very important that they are cleansed before you use them. Crystals, being such good transmitters of energy, tend to pick up all sorts of energies from their surroundings and from those who handle them. This can mean that a crystal contains a mixture of confused energies that need to be cleaned out before you can effectively use it. There are many methods of cleansing a crystal. One method is to place a crystal in a bowl of springwater with a pinch of seasalt dissolved in it, then place it in the sun for an hour. Other methods include smudging (cleansing using smoking herbs such as sage or sweetgrass), placing the crystal under the light of the full moon, or singing to it (see Sound healing, page 184).

Programming a crystal

Once you have cleansed a crystal, it needs programming. This is because a crystal is like a blank television; it needs "tuning in" to get it to work in the way you want it to. Furthermore, crystals can be used in a variety of ways, not just for healing humans, but for working with animals and plants, or for performing ceremonies, or dowsing. By programming a crystal to work in a specific way, you attune its energies and this makes it a much more powerful tool.

All you need to do is hold the crystal in your dominant hand then, with your eyes closed, mentally ask permission to use the crystal for the purpose you require. Unless your intuition calls out a strong "No," you may proceed. Visualize the crystal being filled with all the qualities you require (i.e. healing, balancing, calming etc.). You may see images of animals or other aspects of creation in your mind while doing this. This is quite common and perfectly natural. Continue this visualization

Energizing water with a crystal

This is simply done by placing the crystal of your choice (crystals from the quartz family such as rose quartz, amethyst, or aventurine are ideal) in a clear glass. Fill the glass with springwater and place it in the sun for an hour. The charged water can be stored indefinitely in a blue glass bottle and drunk whenever required.

RIGHT All you need to make energizing crystal water is a glass of springwater and your chosen crystal. Place the crystal in the glass of water and leave in the sunshine for an hour.

for a minimum of 5 minutes and then sit holding your crystal for a further 5 minutes. Your crystal will now be programmed. To reprogram a crystal, first cleanse it in one of the ways described above and then simply program the crystal for its new work.

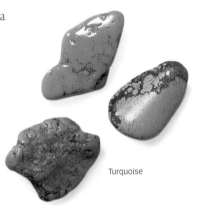

Turquoise

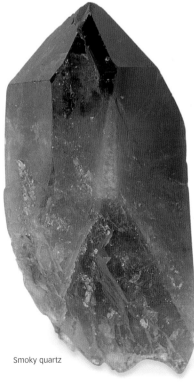

Smoky quartz

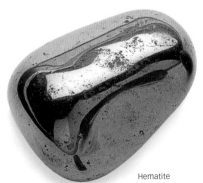

Hematite

The healing properties of crystals

The following is a list of crystals and their healing properties.

AGATE: Calming and stabilizing. Helps in the elimination of negativity.

AMAZONITE: Helps to balance masculine and feminine energies.

AMBER: Used to purify body, mind, and spirit. Has an antiseptic and disinfectant quality.

AMETHYST: A gentle but powerful all around healing stone.

AQUAMARINE: Known as a stone of courage. Good for the throat.

BLOODSTONE: Good for treating all circulatory conditions.

CHRYSOCOLLA: Sometimes called "the crisis stone," helps calm fright and hysteria.

CITRINE: Connected to the sun and so is thought to promote clarity of vision and spiritual enlightenment.

CORAL: Strengthens the skeletal system.

DIAMOND: A strongly protective stone.

EMERALD: Helps dispel negative emotions.

FLUORITE: Helps the body to eliminate toxins and boosts the immune system.

GARNET: Balances sexual energy.

HEMATITE: Is used to treat blood conditions such as anemia.

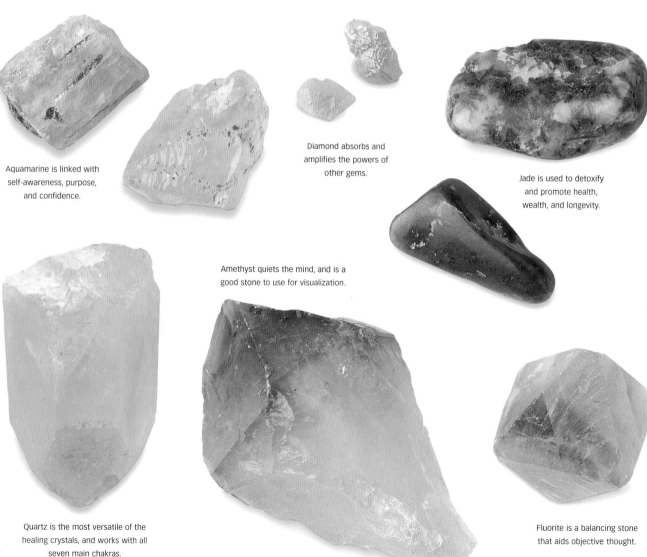

Aquamarine is linked with self-awareness, purpose, and confidence.

Diamond absorbs and amplifies the powers of other gems.

Jade is used to detoxify and promote health, wealth, and longevity.

Amethyst quiets the mind, and is a good stone to use for visualization.

Quartz is the most versatile of the healing crystals, and works with all seven main chakras.

Fluorite is a balancing stone that aids objective thought.

JADE: Helps one to change negative to positive.

JASPER: Used in the treatment of kidney and bladder disorders.

JET: Aids restful sleep and treats migraines.

LAPIS LAZULI: Strengthens the mind and body and attracts wisdom and truth.

MOONSTONE: Balances the emotions.

QUARTZ: Excellent all around healing stone.

ROSE QUARTZ: The heart healer.

SMOKY QUARTZ: Dispels negativity and attracts positivity.

TOURMALINE: Helps to balance the left and right sides of the brain.

TURQUOISE: Strengthens and aligns all the body's energy systems.

Crystals for the chakras

Crystals that resonate with the seven major chakras are:

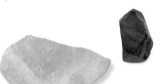

Red stones for the base chakra:
Hematite, red jasper, ruby, garnet, bloodstone, rhodocrosite, red carnelian, spinel, red agate.

Orange stones for the sacral chakra:
Orange carnelian, calcite, amber, topaz.

Yellow stones for the solar plexus chakra: Citrine, yellow jasper, chrysolite, yellow zircon.

Green stones for the heart chakra:
Emerald, green tourmaline, peridot, malachite, amazonite, jade.

Light blue stones for the throat chakra:
Aquamarine, blue lace agate, celestite, turquoise.

Indigo (dark blue) stones for the third eye chakra: Azurite, lapis lazuli, sapphire, sodalite.

Violet stones for the crown chakra:
Amethyst, fluorite, sugilite.

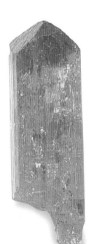

Topaz is a powerful gem that boosts perception and stamina.

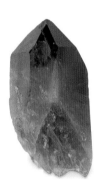

Smoky quartz aids meditation and stimulates the meridians.

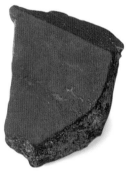

Lapis lazuli opens the mind to higher guidance and intuition.

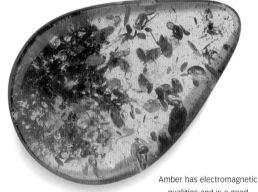

Amber has electromagnetic qualities and is a good mood balancer.

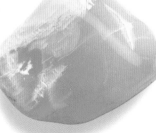

Moonstone helps stress, anxiety, and menstrual imbalances.

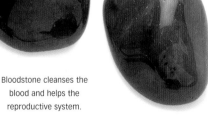

Bloodstone cleanses the blood and helps the reproductive system.

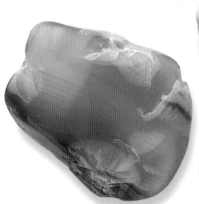

Agate is solid and grounding, and promotes a positive outlook.

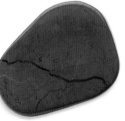

Jasper aids tissue regeneration and general healing.

Emerald strengthens the heart and inspires patience and love.

Gem and crystal elixirs

Gem and crystal elixirs are subtle medicines, healing by the principles of natural resonance. They work at a molecular level, stabilizing any imbalances in the body that can and do cause disease if left uncorrected. Gems are the most potent of the minerals, being the most pure, and so any elixir that is made from a precious gem will have the strongest influence on the human system. Crystal elixirs, or essences as they are generally called, are gentler, but no less effective healers.

Gem and crystal elixirs are made in the same way as flower essences, but while flower essences tend to influence the subtle bodies, mineral elixirs affect the actual bodily structure at a biomolecular level, acting in a similar way to homeopathic remedies. They have the ability to stabilize and ground any imbalances in the body, and can realign the body to its rightful resonance, because they are able to maintain their healing qualities when in contact with disharmonious vibrations. Flower essences are ethereal in nature, while crystal and gem elixirs are based more in the physical world.

Crystals and gems are naturally aligned to the Earth's electromagnetic field, as well as to the human body's electromagnetic structure. A gem or crystal elixir travels through the meridians and eventually rests between the nervous and circulatory systems. From here it affects the biomolecular structures and helps to realign the denser physical, mental, and emotional states with the correct energetic blueprint for that individual's existence.

BELOW Elixirs are made by immersing the crystals or gems in springwater and leaving them in sunshine. The sun's energy pushes the stones' vibrations into the water.

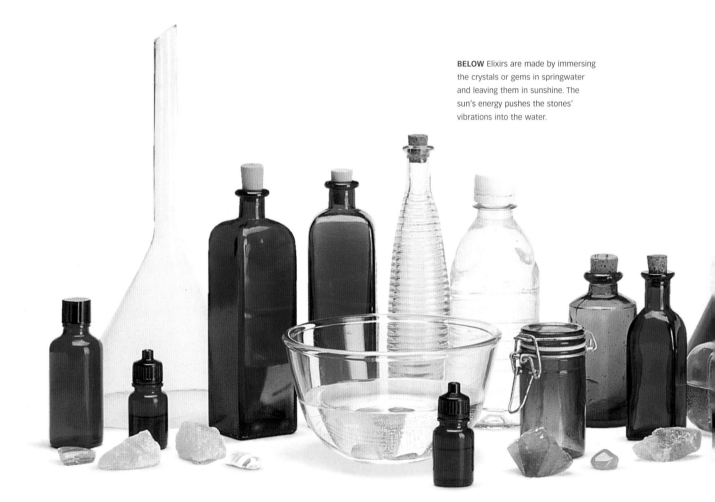

Elixirs and chakras

As a general rule, the color of a gem or crystal indicates which energy center (chakra) it has the strongest influence on. Therefore, an elixir made of a red stone will resonate with the base chakra. Similarly an elixir made with an orange stone will resonate with the belt chakra, a yellow stone with the solar plexus, a green stone with the heart, a light blue stone with the throat, a dark blue stone with the third eye, and a violet or transparent stone with the crown chakra. Placing three drops of a gem or crystal elixir in the palms of your hands, rubbing them together and then resting them on the relevant chakra will bring about the identical balancing effect that placing the same gem or crystal on it would achieve. The elixir of the gem or crystal, when made correctly, carries the blueprint or identity of that stone, and it will have the same healing capacity as the stone in its natural state.

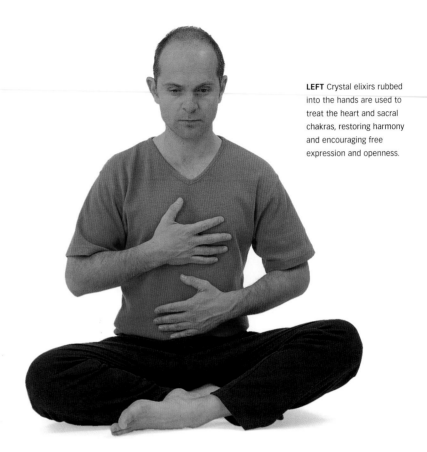

LEFT Crystal elixirs rubbed into the hands are used to treat the heart and sacral chakras, restoring harmony and encouraging free expression and openness.

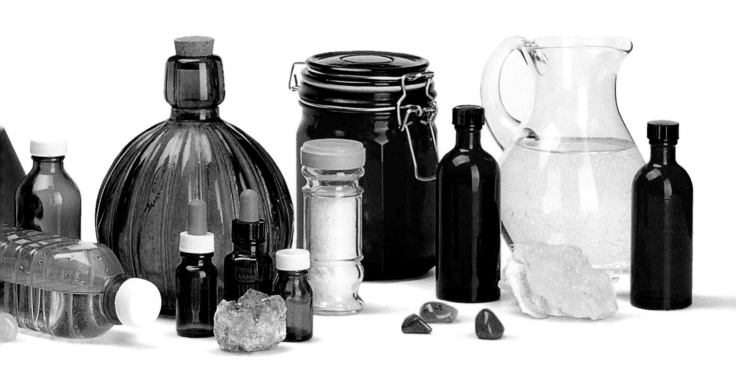

Treating complaints with gem and crystal elixirs

Gem and crystal elixirs are most commonly used to heal physical conditions, or ailments that are well lodged in the physical body. These elixirs are extremely helpful in shifting the body into a high vibration, so that the physical malfunction finds it difficult to maintain its hold. Elixirs can be combined with flower essences to produce a "complete remedy picture" for individual needs, but should not be used with homeopathy because of possible contra-indications.

Elixirs can be administered quite safely to children, elderly, and animals but should not take place of medical care. Consult a qualified vibrational medicine consultant or family doctor with any medical concerns.

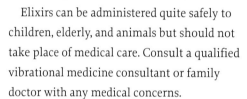

Emerald

Moonstone

Crystal essences and the complaints they help

AMAZONITE: Helps one to align with nature; brings balance.

AMETHYST: Increases clarity and general well-being; treats headaches and nightmares.

AZURITE: Helps arthritic complaints.

BLACK TOURMALINE: Helps to counteract the effects of stress.

CALCITE: Helps maintain healthy bones.

DIAMOND: Helps to increase alignment to one's higher self (good for clearing the mind in confused adolescents).

EMERALD: Promotes peace, harmony, and balance (good for hyperactive children)

MOONSTONE: Treats premenstrual tension and fertility problems.

OBSIDIAN: Soothes stomach upsets (good for motion sickness).

QUARTZ (clear): Helps to strengthen the aura; good after hard, physical work.

STAR SAPPHIRE: Helps to lift depression.

Obsidian

LEFT Gems and crystals are now widely available. Try making your own elixirs and bottling them to preserve their vibrational energy.

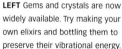

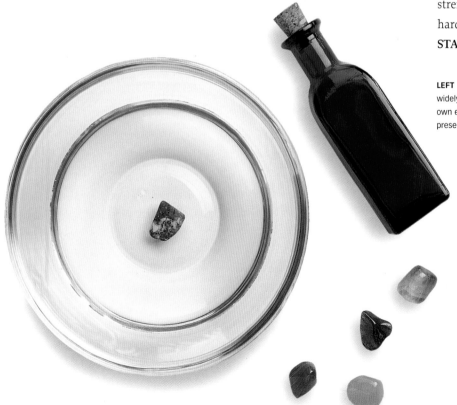

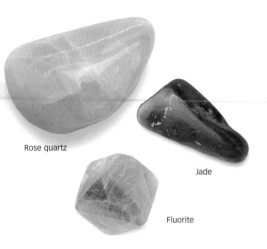

Rose quartz

Jade

Fluorite

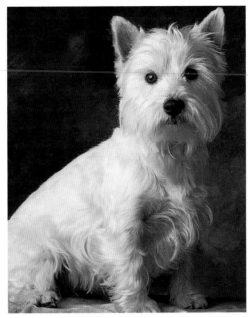

LEFT Animals can benefit from the healing properties of crystal essences, which can improve the condition of their teeth and bones and strengthen their immune system.

Crystal essences for animals

AZURITE: For arthritic conditions.

CALCITE: Treats bone disorders.

FLUORITE: Strengthens teeth (place a few drops in the animal's drinking water).

HERKIMER DIAMOND: Used to support any animal with cancer.

JADE: Supports elderly animals, especially those with weak or dysfunctional kidneys.

LAPIS LAZULI: For bronchial and throat problems.

LODESTONE: Helps with pain relief.

MOSS AGATE: Helps to detoxify the animal's system.

OBSIDIAN: Helps fight infection

ROSE QUARTZ: A safe and gentle all around healing essence for all animals.

In general give a normal adult dose (this is usually written on the bottle) to cats and dogs. For larger animals (such as horses), give twice the adult dose; for smaller animals (such as guinea pigs), give half the adult dose. For birds, fowl, and rodents, place half the adult dose in the daily drinking water.

Remember that these remedies act as a support, not a replacement for professional veterinary advice.

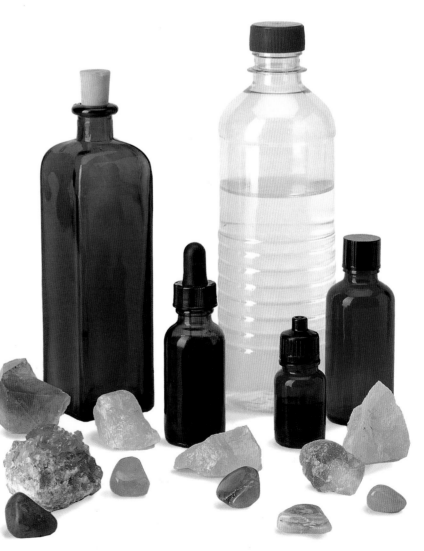

BELOW Using crystals and their elixirs for healing, meditation, and visualization will gradually attune you to the energies surrounding you.

Flowers and plants

Since the dawn of time, humankind has formed a close bond with flowers and plants. Early Neanderthal graves show strong evidence that our Stone Age relatives covered the bodies of their dead with fragrant herbs at the time of burial. No doubt these early hunter-gatherers noticed that certain animals ate specific plants for health purposes. The chamois deer, for instance, will eat spurges if bitten by a snake (a plant belonging to the genus, *Euphorbia*), which gives it violent diarrhea. Wolves eat the root of the bistort for similar reasons. The hunter-gatherers would have also noticed that animals used plants for external medicine as well. The muskrat, if wounded, will coat its wounds with the resin from pine trees as an antiseptic. This knowledge would have been accumulated and passed down from generation to generation via the female (wise woman) line from grandmother to mother to daughter and so on.

ABOVE Hippocrates drew from the work of his predecessors to found scientific medicine.

About 5,000 years ago in China, the *Pen Ts'ao* herbal was written. This listed the use of many plants and flowers for healing. In Egypt, medical papyri from 1500 B.C.E. record over 260 medicinal plants, and in Assyria ancient clay tablets record 250 similar herbs.

In India, an ancient Hindu text, called the *Atharavaveda*, dating from the second century B.C.E. records details of many herbal and folk remedies for various ills. In the early part of the Common Era (C.E. 0–700) two medical and herbal works, the *Charaka Samhita* and *Susruta Samhita*, were written down, and now form the foundations of the Indian tradition of Ayurvedic medicine.

The founders of herbalism in the West

Perhaps the most famous of all herbalists is Hippocrates. This great Greek philosopher was born around 400 B.C.E. and founded a school of medicine that gave the West much of its medical and herbal knowledge.

Theophrastus, regarded as the "Father of Botany," was born around 372 B.C.E. on the Greek island of Lesbos. He provided a new understanding of plants in the West. Pliny the Elder, born around C.E. 23, wrote some 37 volumes on natural history, including details of many medicinal plants. The Greek physician Dioscorides, who lived during the first century C.E., produced the West's first *Materia Medica*

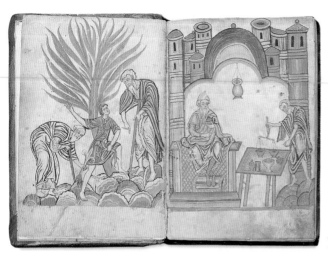

ABOVE Herbalists dig plants from a medicinal garden and prepare remedies in this medieval version of a manuscript by the Greek physician Pedanius Dioscorides.

detailing more than 500 medicinal plants. Galen, regarded as the "Father of Pharmacy," was born around C.E. 130 in Pergamum in Greece. Some of his herbal recipes are still used today by modern pharmacists.

English herbalism

The first known herbal to appear in the English language was written by Richard Banckes in 1526, although it is thought to have been based on earlier herbal manuals. It was followed in 1597 by *Gerard's Herbal*, which contained 1,630 lavishly illustrated pages detailing many medicinal herbs and herbal preparations. In 1629 an herbalist, John Parkinson, published an herbal manual called *Paradisi in Sole* and the *London Dispensatory* followed this in 1651 written by Nicholas Culpeper, the famous herbalist, astrologer, and doctor. John Ray published his *Catalogus Plantorum Angliae* in 1670 and John Pechey published the last of the real *English Herbals* in 1694.

In modern times, the most renowned herbal, the *Modern Herbal*, written by Mary Grieve and Hilda Leyel was published in 1931. It has become the main reference manual of many of today's working herbalists.

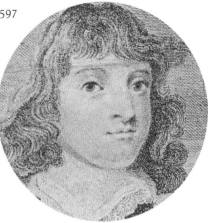

ABOVE Nicholas Culpeper (1616–54) practiced in Spitalfields, in London. His bestselling books soon became the most famous publications on herbalism in the English language.

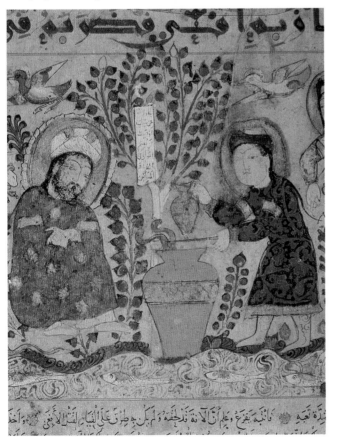

LEFT A doctor uses plants to treat poisoning in a 12th-century Arabian book of antidotes. Arabian herbal lore was mainly developed by monks experimenting with ingredients inside monasteries. The Arabian medical tradition kept the physician's role separate from the role of the pharmacist. The physician diagnosed and the pharmacist created the remedy.

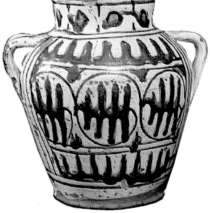

ABOVE This apothecary storage jar, c.1425–50, was once used to store herbal oils for mixing into creams and ointments that were used to treat skin disorders.

The flower essences of Edward Bach

Edward Bach (1886–1936) was a highly successful and well-respected physician in London. However, he became more interested in the people he treated than in the diseases they manifested. He discovered that the root causes of many diseases were imbalanced emotions and he set about creating a series of flower remedies to treat these causes. The results he achieved were remarkable and often miraculous. His 38 remedies have formed the foundation of all modern flower remedy use. Each remedy treats negative emotions, allowing the patient to change these emotions into positive ones. They are subtle, yet very powerful catalysts or tools for transformation.

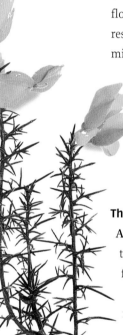

ABOVE Gorse, *Ulex europaeus,* a flower remedy for reassurance.

The Bach remedies

AGRIMONY: For those who suffer inner torture, which they try to hide behind a facade of cheerfulness.

ASPEN: For fears of unknown origin and for apprehension or foreboding.

BEECH: For those who are arrogant, critical, and intolerant of others.

CENTAURY: For those who, due to weakness of will, allow themselves to be imposed upon and for those who have difficulty saying "no."

CERATO: For those who are easily influenced or misguided and actively seek the advice of others while doubting their own judgement.

CHERRY PLUM: For a fear of mental collapse, desperation, loss of control, and for violent rages.

CHESTNUT BUD: For those people who continually make the same mistakes.

CHICORY: For overpossessiveness or attention seeking.

CLEMATIS: For indifference, inattentiveness, dreaminess, or absent-mindedness.

CRAB APPLE: For those who feel unclean or ashamed. For self-disgust and housepride.

ELM: For those who are temporarily overcome by responsibility or inadequacy although they are normally very capable.

GENTIAN: For the despondent and those easily discouraged.

GORSE: For extreme hopelessness.

HEATHER: For those who are obsessed with their own troubles and experiences.

HOLLY: For those who are consumed by jealousy, hatred, envy, or the desire for revenge.

HONEYSUCKLE: For those who are homesick or dwell in the past.

HORNBEAM: For procrastination.

IMPATIENS: For impatience and irritability.

LARCH: For despondency due to a lack of self-confidence. For those who expect to fail.

MIMULUS: For fear of known things, shyness, and timidity.

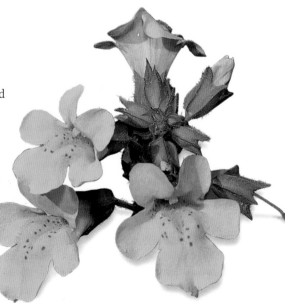

RIGHT Monkey-flower, *Mimulus luteus,* for courage.

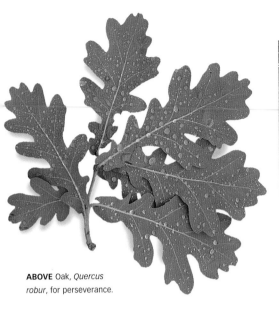

ABOVE Oak, *Quercus robur*, for perseverance.

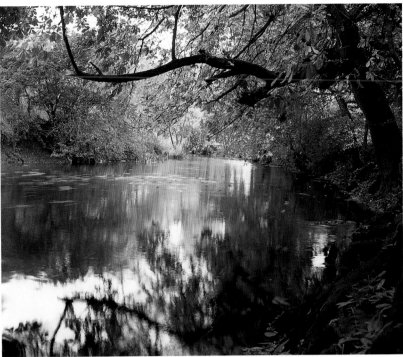

MUSTARD: For deep gloom that descends for no known reason but can lift just as suddenly; for feelings of melancholy.

OAK: For those who struggle on in illness and against adversity despite setbacks.

OLIVE: For exhaustion.

PINE: For feelings of guilt and unworthiness.

RED CHESTNUT: For excessive fear and overcaring for others.

ROCK ROSE: For terror, extreme fear, or panic.

ROCK WATER: For those who are hard on themselves, rigid-minded, and self-denying.

SCLERANTHUS: For uncertainty, indecision, and vacillation.

STAR OF BETHLEHEM: For the effects of bad news or fright following an accident.

SWEET CHESTNUT: For the anguish of those who have reached the limits of endurance and absolute dejection.

VERVAIN: For overenthusiasm, overeffort, and straining; fanaticism.

VINE: For those with dominating personalities who are inflexible, ambitious, arrogant, and proud.

WALNUT: Helps with adjustments and transitions.

WATER VIOLET: For those who are proud, reserved, or "superior."

WHITE CHESTNUT: For worry and persistent unwanted thoughts.

WILD OAT: For those who are trying to determine their path in life.

WILD ROSE: For resignation, apathy, and those who make little effort for improvement.

WILLOW: For resentment and bitterness.

RESCUE REMEDY: This is an all-purpose emergency remedy made from a combination of cherry plum, clematis, impatiens, rock rose, and Star of Bethlehem.

ABOVE The balance of nature captured in Dr. Edward Bach's flower remedies steadies the emotions.

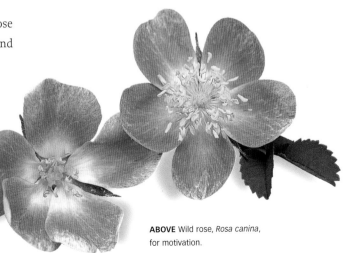

ABOVE Wild rose, *Rosa canina*, for motivation.

Flower essences

For many years the Bach Flower Remedies stood alone, but in the last 20 years many of the original flower essences that were commonly used by ancient cultures have been rediscovered. These essences continue to be researched – so much so that today we are experiencing a resurgence of the use of flower essences with over 30 different families of remedy gathered from least 50 countries.

Many diverse and exotic blooms hailing from Hawaii, Alaska, the Australian Bush, the Amazonian rain forest, from the valley of the flowers in the Himalayas, to the desert plains of Texas, and Arizona, make up this growing repertoire of healing flowers. These floral essences when ingested in drop form, or put on the wrists or chakra points, rekindle a feeling of well-being and balance to body, mind, and spirit. Some bring relief from stress, anxiety, and fear while others release deep-seated behavioral patterns. There are now remedies that help with acutely physical problems, from migraine headaches and hormonal problems to boosting the immune system in order to inhibit viral attack.

The flowers' power to heal is thought to reside in their special vibrational qualities. Each flower is packed with its own unique energy in characteristics which it

BELOW African violet, *Saintpaulia*, essence helps overcome shyness and encourages openness and interaction with others.

BELOW Poppy essences have been used to recall and release memories of past lives and initiate forgiveness.

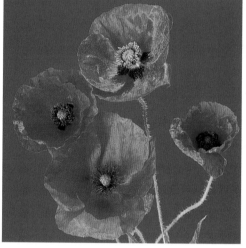

emanates. The flower's essence acts as a catalyst to bring our energies back into balance with our own original blueprint of perfect health. They have the capacity to do this, as the vibrations they emit are at the frequencies that are closely matched to those of our own subtle energies. They work to realign and pull the

ABOVE Essences distilled from tropical orchids have been known to help addictive behavior, leading to a more intuitive way of life directed by the heart.

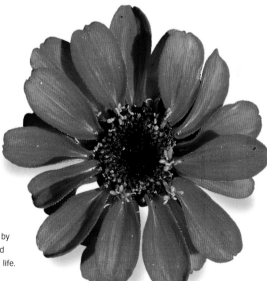

RIGHT Zinnia essence treats overseriousness and repression by bringing out the "inner child" and giving a sense of perspective on life.

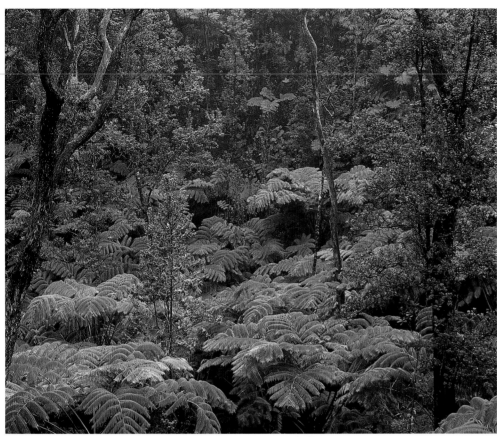

subtle anatomy back into order so the self-healing process can begin. Acting in a specific way, they travel to the areas that are in most need of attention and these areas of vibrational imbalance literally soak up the essence's healing energy like a sponge.

The flower remedies not only have a particular resonance with the chakras, meridians, aura, and subtle bodies, but also directly affect the physical body. Furthermore, flowers that were often held to be sacred and had spiritual significance when used in ceremonies (i.e. lotus, rose and orchid), in essence form are used for tapping into the realms of the spirit and aiding spiritual advancement and empowerment. Flower essences help us to come back into perfect alignment with ourselves, reminding the body how it should be, and helping us to fulfill our true destiny in life.

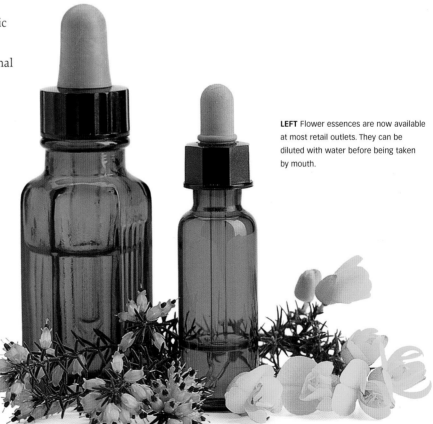

Traditional Herbalism

Traditional herbalism has roots that go back to the Stone Age. Throughout the world, herbal knowledge has been passed down from generation to generation through wise women, shamans, medicine men and women, and witch doctors. It is still used as the primary form of healing in many tribal cultures including Aboriginal, African, Native American, South American, and Celtic. All these cultures have one common belief: that belief is that all plants have an "energy" or "spirit" that can be communicated with. Many practitioners still use trance states or meditation to communicate with these energies. They receive much or all of their instruction as to the correct dosage and preparation of the herb from the plant itself.

The original herbalists

In times past, before the written word, a local tribal healer would have to rely on his or her intuition and their ability to talk with nature to exact healing on a sick person. The ill person would seek the advice of the healer who, after diagnosing the problem, would go out into the wilds and collect herbs according

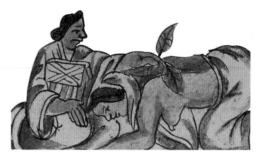

ABOVE Aztec manuscripts display their faith in plant medicines. This illustration shows a midwife administering herbs to a woman to ease her discomfort after childbirth.

to intuition and "calling." This may sound incredible but a similar method was utilized by Dr. Edward Bach in the preparation of his 38 flower remedies. Dr. Bach would often manifest a negative mental state himself and then find the cure by picking flowers and placing them on his tongue. The energy of the correct plant to treat those symptoms would bring Dr. Bach almost instant relief.

The plants used would often not contain recognized therapeutic ingredients and yet their overall energy would have a direct effect on the underlying emotional cause of the illness. Exactly the same practice is followed by many shamans, wise women, and medicine people throughout the world.

Medical herbalism and traditional herbalism

Medical herbalism tends to treat symptoms using herbs in place of drugs. Although many medical herbalists attempt to treat holistically, many others still treat only symptomatically. Traditional herbalism, on the other hand, treats only the underlying imbalances. It relies on direct communication with the plant spirits to gain knowledge that is not normally available to a practitioner. Most traditional herbalists also believe that any ecosystem contains all the herbs necessary to treat all of the imbalances that manifest in that

ABOVE Catmint (top), *Nepeta cataria*, is used in medicinal teas to treat colds and fever. Rue (below), *Ruta graveolens*, yields oil used to aid digestion.

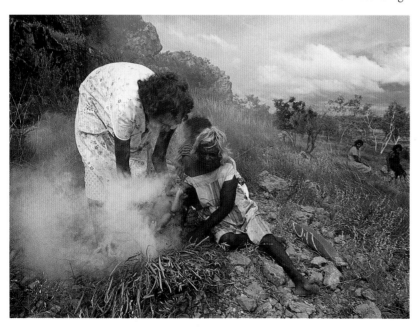

LEFT Herbal incense fills the air as women light a fire (a symbol of human power) at an Aboriginal ceremony, welcoming the newborn to the physical world.

ecosystem. This means that a traditional herbalist treating in England would generally only use English herbs. Likewise an Aboriginal healer would only use Australian herbs.

LEFT A Chinese goddess of medicine. Her existence demonstrates the importance in Eastern philosophies of maintaining a healthy body and mind.

Finding out about traditional herbalism

Traditional herbalism has been suppressed in many countries by the authorities and the church both in the past and sometimes in the present. There are, however, wise men and women throughout the world who still retain this knowledge. It still forms an integral part of shamanic practice in most cultures including those mentioned earlier. It is a form of medicine that recognizes that we are all connected to each other and to creation by the web of life. It is a type of herbalism that everyone can benefit from because as you discover your place and connections on the web of life, you will naturally find the path to health, happiness, and fulfillment. If you want to discover more about the herbalism of your land, look at the early, pre-Christian, native practices of the people who originated in your land. As you discover more about your roots and you will uncover more of this hidden knowledge. Plants and flowers have many things to teach us over and beyond the symptomatic relief of our various ailments.

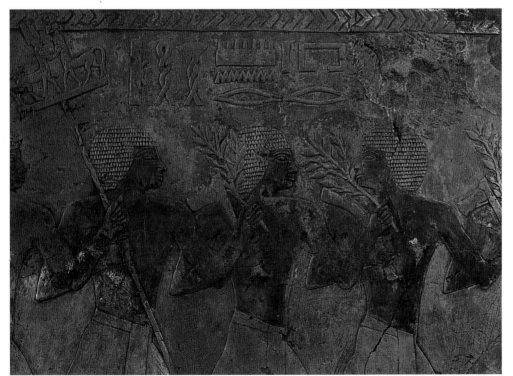

LEFT The Egyptians were practitioners of herbal medicine. A relief from the funerary temple of Queen Hatshepsut shows a visit to Punt, a place famous for its incense. The queen's servants return laden with herbs from its plants and bushes.

Aromatherapy

Aromatherapy involves the treatment of illness using highly concentrated aromatic oils, known as essential oils, extracted from plants. It is thought to have originated in ancient China, although the Egyptians were also known to have experimented with aromatic oils as early as 1550 B.C.E.

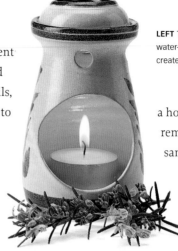

LEFT Three drops of oil in the water-filled tray of a burner create a good aroma.

The modern-day pioneer of aromatherapy was a French chemist called Professor René Gattefosse. He discovered the healing power of lavender oil by accident when he plunged his hand into a vat of the oil after badly burning himself. To his surprise the pain stopped and the burn healed, leaving neither blister nor scar. He went on to use various oils to treat sick and injured soldiers during the First World War.

Later, a French doctor, Dr. Jean Valnet, built on Gattefosse's work using oils in the treatment of cancer, diabetes, tuberculosis, and a host of other ailments with remarkable success. At the same time, Marguerite Maury, a French biochemist and beautician developed such techniques as massage and various skin-care treatments using essential oils. Today aromatherapy is an established therapy that can help to treat many illnesses, including depression, headache, arthritis, rheumatism, joint pain, insomnia, skin disorders, and stress.

Methods of aromatherapy

There are many ways that essential oils can be used to treat illnesses:

INHALATION: Particularly good for sinus and breathing problems caused by colds, the flu, and hay fever. A few drops of oil can be placed on a handkerchief, a pillow, or evaporated in a bowl of hot water.

VAPORIZATION: This is an ideal way to cleanse rooms of infection. A few drops of lavender or tea-tree oil evaporated in an oil burner can help to disinfect a room of germs. The simplest way to evaporate oils is by placing a few drops onto a cotton ball and then placing the ball on a hot radiator. You can also purchase vaporizing rings to place on lightbulbs.

WATER AS A CARRIER: Aromatic baths can be used to relax the body and to aid certain problems such as aches and pains, insomnia, and arthritis. Compresses containing a few drops of lavender or peppermint oil can help to relieve headaches and migraines.

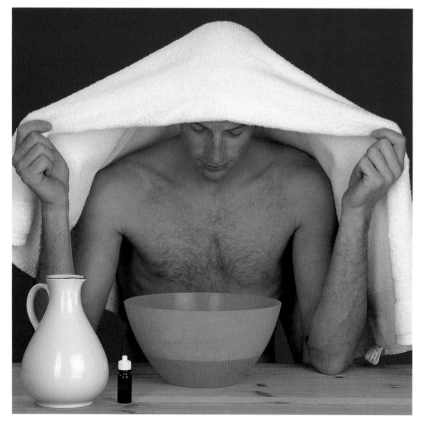

BELOW An aromatherapy inhalation made with a few drops of basil (uplifting) or hyssop (a decongestant) will help breathing problems.

OILS AND LOTIONS AS CARRIERS: Massage is the most popular of all aromatherapy treatments. Essential oils are dissolved in a carrier oil such as grapeseed or sweet almond oil. The essential oils are absorbed through the skin during and after the massage. Usually up to 10–20 drops in total of a single or several essential oils are mixed in 2 fl oz (50ml) of carrier oil.

The characteristics of essential oils

Each oil has a set of characteristics that dictate its therapeutic use. For instance, bergamot is uplifting and relaxing, while lemon is stimulating and refreshing. Combining oils can alter their therapeutic natures and the correct blending of oils is a very skilled technique. Having said that, when used with common sense, essential oils have been proven to be safe for personal use by adults and children alike. If you are using oils at home, use only high quality oils from a specialist supplier. Do not be afraid to blend oils; many aromatherapy oils actually work better when combined with other essential oils. Never apply undiluted essential oils directly to the skin except when treating burns (use undiluted lavender oil) or bites, minor cuts and stings (use undiluted tea-tree oil). Finally, do not swallow oils unless directed to by a qualified practitioner. The chart on page 174 shows the most commonly used essential oils, their effects, and uses.

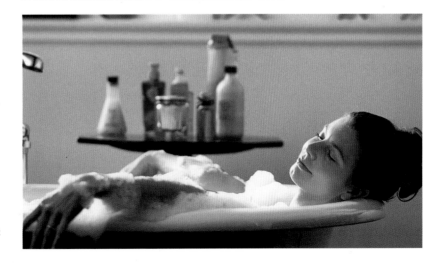

RIGHT Try adding a few drops of essential oil to a warm bath: lavender or patchouli for deep relaxation, rosemary or bergamot for invigoration.

The effects and uses of aromatherapy oils

OIL	EFFECTS	USES
Basil	Uplifting, refreshing	Bronchitis, depression, earache, nausea, breathing problems, digestive disorders, stress, mental fatigue, insomnia.
Bergamot	Uplifting, refreshing, relaxing	Herpes, ulcers, sore throat, fevers, depression, scabies, gallstones, psoriasis.
Black pepper	Stimulating	Cold, congestion, constipation, diarrhea, dysentery, gas, food poisoning, toothache, loss of appetite, and vertigo.
Chamomile	Soothing, relaxing	Allergies, boils, colic, depression, earache, fevers, headache, hysteria, insomnia, menopausal problems, teething pains, vaginitis.
Camphor	Cooling, stimulating	Acne, bronchitis, bruises, burns, colds, gout, inflammation, insomnia, nervous tension, rheumatism, shock, sprains.
Cedarwood	Sedative, antiseptic	Acne, anxiety, congestion, coughs, cystitis, skin diseases, urinary tract infections.
Clary sage	Warming, relaxing	Boils, convulsions, depression, gas, frigidity, hypertension, impotence, kidney disorders, menstrual problems.
Cypress	relaxing, refreshing	Asthma, diarrhea, hemorrhoids, the flu, liver disorders, menopausal problems, varicose veins.
Eucalyptus	Stimulating, clears the head	Breathing disorders, colds, congestion, cough, cystitis, diabetes, fevers, headaches, malaria, measles, scarlet fever, skin ulcers.
Fennel	Eases gas and stomach pains	Colic, constipation, gas, hiccups, insufficient milk (in nursing mothers), kidney stones, nausea, obesity, vomiting.
Frankincense	Relaxing, rejuvenating	Bronchitis, carbuncles, cystitis, skin disorders, stress, ulcers, wounds.
Geranium	Refreshing, relaxing	Burns, depression, dermatitis, ringworm, shingles, sore throats, ulcers (internal and external), urinary infections, varicose veins, wounds.
Hyssop	Decongestant, tonic	Breathing problems, bruises, eczema, gas, general poor health, rheumatism, whooping cough.
Jasmine (absolute, not pure oil)	Relaxing, soothing	Apathy, anxiety, depression, frigidity, impotence, skin disorders.

OIL	EFFECTS	USES
Juniper	Refreshing, relaxing, stimulating	Arteriosclerosis, cirrhosis, dermatitis, eczema, general poor health, gout, rheumatoid arthritis, ulcers (external).
Lavender (good for children)	Refreshing, relaxing	Abscess, asthma, boils, bronchitis, burns, carbuncles, colic, congestion, conjunctivitis, cystitis, depression, dermatitis, diarrhea, diphtheria, dyspepsia, earache, eczema, epilepsy, fainting, gas, halitosis, headache, hysteria, insomnia, sunstroke, and many, many more.
Lemon	Refreshing, stimulating	Acne, poor circulation, high blood pressure.
Marjoram	Warming, strengthening	Arthritis, cramps, constipation, gas, headache, hysteria, insomnia, migraine, nervous tension, tic.
Melissa (Lemon balm)	Uplifting, calming	Allergies, depression, dysentery, fevers, menstrual problems, palpitations, nervous tension, shock, sterility (in women).
Peppermint	Cooling, refreshing	Any lung disorder, fainting, mental fatigue, migraines, motion sickness, nausea, ringworm, scabies, shock, toothache, vertigo, vomiting.
Rosemary (good for children)	Invigorating, refreshing	Colds, depression, fainting, hair loss, headaches, migraines, nervousness, palpitations, whooping cough.
Sage	Improves circulation	Poor circulation, rheumatism, viral infections.
Sandalwood	Calming, cleansing	Cough, hiccups, muzziness in the head, nausea.
Tea tree	Antiseptic, cleansing	Athlete's foot, coughs, colds, cuts, sore throats, wounds, yeast infections.

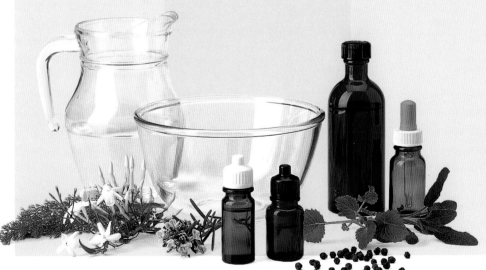

LEFT Mix essential oils into different combinations to find out which aromas appeal to you. Popular oils such as lavender, geranium, and basil are relatively cheap; jasmine and sandalwood cost a little more.

Homeopathy

Homeopathy is a system of medicine developed by Samuel Hahnemann, a German physician who practiced during the early part of the 18th century. The word "homeopathy" comes from two Greek words *omio* meaning "the same" and *pathos* meaning "suffering." This reflects the fundamental law of homeopathy, *simila similibus curentur* or "let like be cured with like."

Homeopathic remedies are made from substances (plants, minerals, and animal products) that have been potentized. This technique involves highly diluting the substance and "succussing" (vigorously shaking) the dilution. A substance that has the potential to make you ill in its raw state, has the potential to cure when potentized. Some potentized remedies, such as arsenic, are fatal in their raw state but when potentized can produce remarkable healing. Homeopathy, like most medical systems, uses symptoms as clues to understanding the patient's disease. However, homeopathy looks at the whole patient and symptoms that may seem unconnected are not treated separately, but form part of an overall pattern of disharmony. The homeopath will look for a remedy that most reflects all the manifesting symptoms.

Homeopathy has a detailed medical philosophy based on observation of how the human body becomes ill and cures itself. Hahnemann originally wrote these ideas down in a book, which he called *The*

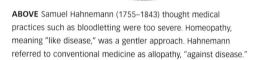

ABOVE Samuel Hahnemann (1755–1843) thought medical practices such as bloodletting were too severe. Homeopathy, meaning "like disease," was a gentler approach. Hahnemann referred to conventional medicine as allopathy, "against disease."

Organon. Today the work of Hahnemann continues to be built on with new observations of patients being recorded and new remedies being developed. Homeopathy tempers contemporary philosophies and modern scientific theory with sound clinical observation and the basic principles of homeopathy as taught by Hahnemann.

Who can homeopathy help?

Homeopathy claims to be able to treat all illness, but the pattern of treatment varies from individual to individual because the patient is treated holistically. This means that a thin, nervous patient with a cold will be treated differently to an outgoing, overweight person with a cold. The cold is regarded as only one of a whole range of disharmonious patterns within the patient. One of the problems with homeopathy is that there are so many thousands of different remedies to treat many varied illnesses that it can take

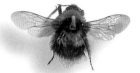

LEFT Apis, a homeopathic remedy for hot, swollen bites and stings, hives and cystitis, is made from whole bees. It reduces inflammation and burning pain.

THE LAWS OF SIMILARITY

The word Homeopathy is a combination of two Greek words: *omoio* which means like or similar and *pathos* which means suffering. During the fifth century B.C.E., the Greek physician Hippocrates had observed that there were two methods of healing, by "contraries" or by "similars." Toward the end of the eighteenth century Samuel Hahnemann took this observation a step further by discovering that it was possible to treat a someone showing symptoms of a particular disease with substances which would cause symptoms of that disease in a healthy person. Hahnemann named this principle the Law of Similars and went on to develop this principle of "let like by cured by like" by researching a wide range of homeopathic treatments. He published his work in *The Organon*, a book which is still regarded as the definitive work by many homeopaths today.

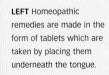

LEFT Euphrasia or common eyebright soothes sore eyes.

LEFT Homeopathic remedies are made in the form of tablets which are taken by placing them underneath the tongue.

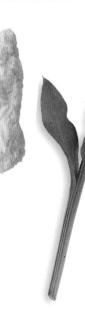

ABOVE Poisonous Belladonna or Deadly Nightshade, when taken homepoathically, cures headaches and fever.

several treatments using different remedies to treat different levels of illness. Homeopathic treatment requires patience and persistence if a cure is to be found.

How to find a homeopath

Choosing a homeopath is similar to seeking any professional advice and positive personal recommendation is one of the most valuable sources of information. Meeting with a homeopath to talk about their relevant experience and how they practice is also useful. Most professional homeopaths undertake a comprehensive 3–4 year training. They then go on to practice under supervision and finally apply to a professional society that insures professional standards are maintained.

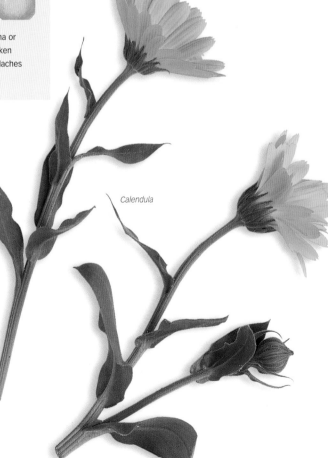

Calendula

BELOW *Hypericum* (St. John's Wort) is taken to remedy nerve pain, *Hepar Sulfur* (sulfur) treats colds and hypersensitivity and Calendula (pot marigold) is an antiseptic for cuts and wounds.

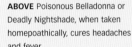

Sulfur

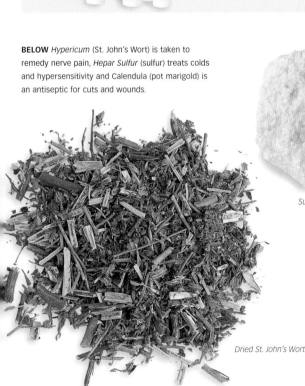

Dried St. John's Wort

color, sound, and light

"The vital spirits of humankind, tuned to the tone of heaven and Earth, express all the tremors of heaven and Earth, just as several cithars (a musical stringed instrument), all tuned on gong (to C tonic), all vibrate when the note gong sounds. The fact of harmony between heaven and Earth and humankind does not come from a physical union, from a direct action; it comes from a tuning on the same note producing vibrations in unison...In the universe nothing happens by chance, there is no spontaneity; all is influence and harmony accord answering accord." Dong Zhongzu, a second century Chinese philosopher

Everything in the universe vibrates. Color, light, and sound are manifestations of that vibration. When something vibrates at a certain frequency, it emits light. If it vibrates at another frequency it emits sound. Pure notes and pure colors are harmonious and pleasing to the ear and eye. If you could see an illness in terms of color, it would be a mass of dark or discordant colors. Likewise, if you could hear an illness, it would be perceived as a jumble of inharmonious noise. The therapists who work with color, light, and sound recognize that inharmonious and discordant vibrations can cause illness and disease. They seek to use the harmonious vibrations of color, light, or sound to restore the balance within their patient. It is as if the colors and sounds offer the body a harmonious pattern to match its own energies to.

"The spirit within us is the only all-powerful doctor, and the only true panacea is to submit oneself to it." Sri Aurobindo, an Indian mystic

The power of color, light, and sound

To fully understand the power of color, light, and sound, one has to experience it firsthand. As you walk through life, start to become aware of the colors, sounds, and light around you. How do they influence you? Do some colors or sounds make you feel uncomfortable and do others make you feel warm and

LEFT Nature's vibrant colors are available to everyone. The deep yellow of sunflowers inspires and stimulates. In color therapy, yellow treats skin disorders and arthritic conditions.

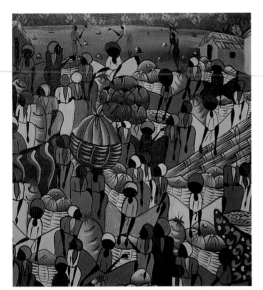

LEFT The vitality of an ethnic market is reflected in its colors. In the West, our lack of color shows a loss of connection with our natural surroundings.

nourished? Begin to perceive the subtle vibrations that emanate from all matter. This will inevitably lead you to perceive the subtle vibrations emanating from your "soul." These are guiding vibrations that can help you on your journey to discover happiness, health, and fulfillment.

Every thought you have, positive or negative, sends energy out to the universe. Those vibrations attract other vibrations to themselves that return back to the source (you!) which means, "as you sow, so shall you reap." If you think negative thoughts, you will attract negativity to yourself. If you think only positive, beautiful thoughts, your life will become more beautiful and harmonious. Your very thoughts are influencing the pattern of your life. Take full responsibility for your every thought, word, and action because they each transmit real vibrations. Once you do this, you will begin to understand the power that is latent within you. You have the ability to influence the vibrations you send out and those that you attract.

All energies and vibrations have their origin in the spiritual realm. This is often why we do not understand the reasons why we are attracting certain energies into our lives. Everything comes to teach. Once you truly understand this concept, you will be able to concentrate on learning all that you need to make your life happy, healthy, and fulfilled rather than fighting the energies created by your own powers of thought.

ABOVE The clear, harmonious sounds of a stringed instrument are drawn out by the strong vibrations caused by the player's bow.

Color Healing

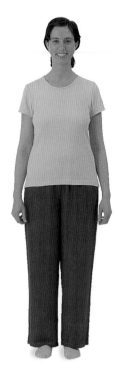

We are constantly bathed in color, from the moment we are born until the day we disincarnate. Much of our lives is strongly influenced by color. In our homes, work, clothing, car, everything is color. We have color codes such as "red for danger," "green for go," and so on. Color even pervades our description of moods such as "green with envy," "feeling blue," and "seeing red."

We all form a lifelong relationship with colors, choosing our favorite and least favorite ones, using color to change our moods (i.e. putting on different colored clothing) and so on. The world of nature shows us the richest and most varied range of ever-changing colors. Spring, summer, winter, and fall each have their own colors, which give us unconscious messages that our body responds to, allowing us to adjust to the changing seasons.

ABOVE Yellow is associated with the power of thought. Blue is associated with peace and tranquility.

Our responses to color

Generally, red tends to be stimulating to the body. Prisoners kept in red cells are much more prone to violent outbursts than those kept in pale blue cells. Rooms that are painted red appear smaller than blue ones, and prolonged exposure to the color red increases blood pressure and aggressiveness ("a red rag to a bull"). Blue on the other hand is generally much more calming. Exposure to this color relaxes the body and actually lowers blood pressure. The power of color to influence our lives for good or ill has been known in the East for thousands of years and its acceptance in the West is growing with the ever-expanding interest in energy and energy healing.

BELOW Fall reds and browns are earth colors. They energize the body and have a grounding effect. Yellow, the color of the sun, stimulates the mind.

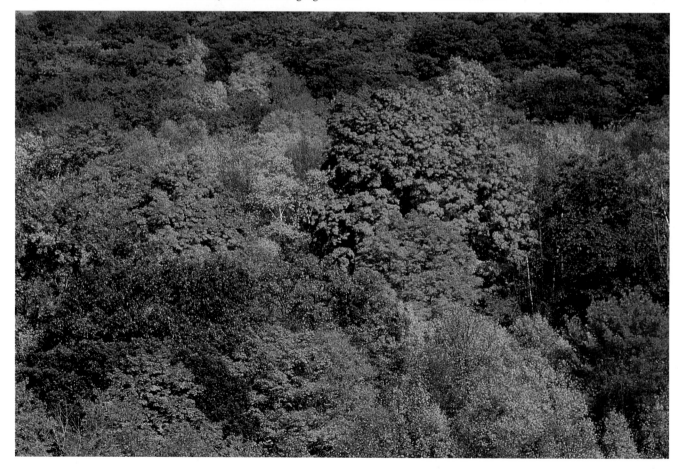

The power of color

Red is the color of dynamic and expressive energy. It is often linked to rage, anger, and aggression but this is only one aspect of the color red. Red is a stimulating and exciting color that acts as an amplifier of emotions. Red will only amplify the emotions that are already existing within us. If you are balanced, red will not make you angry. Red fuels expression rather than creating aggression. Red is a very warming color and is used in color healing to bring warmth to areas of the body that are cold and stiff. Red increases red blood-cell production, it encourages sluggish menstruation, and stimulates the autonomic nervous system. It is also the color linked to the base chakra and to primal sexual energy. All this makes red a powerful color in treating arthritis, rheumatism, lumbago, sciatica, impotence, frigidity, and general lethargy.

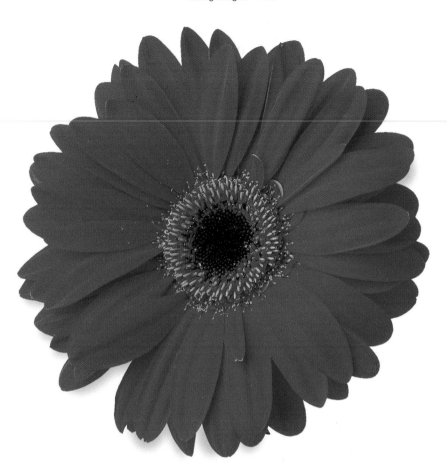

ABOVE Red is an energizing color. It is a symbol of masculine energy, and in some traditions this color denotes supernatural or solar power.

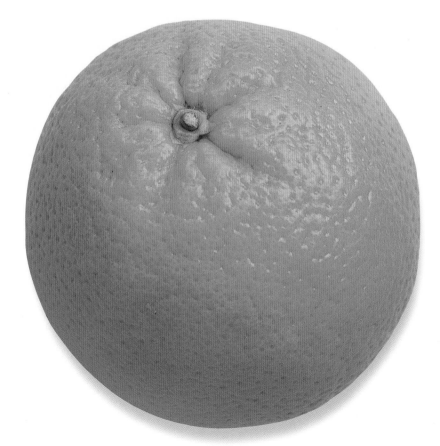

Orange combines the energies of reproduction with those of intellectual stimulation. It aids digestion (both physical and mental), helping absorption and assimilation. It too is a warming color and it helps to increase oxygen levels in the body by stimulating the breathing. Orange is linked to the belt chakra and is used by color healers to relieve menstrual cramps, release gas, draw out boils, and bring abscesses to a head. Orange is a color that depresses the parathyroid and stimulates the thyroid. This action is particularly useful for nursing mothers because it stimulates milk production in the breasts.

LEFT Orange is warming and stimulating, and is associated with love and happiness. It is also a symbol of the feminine energy of creation.

Yellow is the color of the intellect and intelligence. Its vibration acts directly on the mind, stimulating and balancing it, making yellow particularly useful in the treatment of mental problems. In many cultures yellow flowers are always brought to the bed of a sick person, perhaps acknowledging the fact that all illness starts in the mind. Yellow reinforces self-confidence and promotes courage. It improves assimilation within the body and energizes the liver, gallbladder, lymphatic system, the eyes, and the ears. It is used by color healers to help to dissolve uric and lactic acid crystals and to loosen lime deposits around joints in the treatment of gout, rheumatism, and arthritis. Holding a yellow flower or crystal is very energizing when you are feeling emotionally or mentally drained.

Green is the color of intuition and wisdom. It marks the point of balance between the stimulating and warming reds, oranges and yellows and the relaxing and cooling blues, indigos, and purples. Because of its position in the middle of the color spectrum, it is a powerful color for balancing the energies. It is also the primary color of nature and is linked to the heart chakra, which is at the center of our being. Without love, there is no life and the color green vibrates with the energy of love and life. Take a walk in the country and you will be able to feel this wonderful, balancing energy. Green stimulates the pituitary gland and aids cell growth and regeneration. Color healers use it to treat open wounds, sores, bruises, and scars and to help the body dissolve blood clots and fight infection.

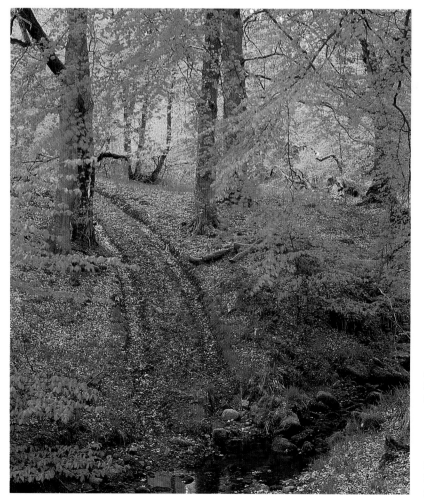

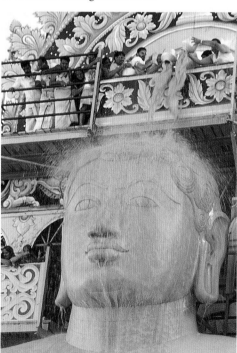

ABOVE Yellow turmeric powder symbolizing the sun is scattered by devotees of the Hindu god Shiva at the Indian festival of Somavati Amavasya.

LEFT Green is the color of life and a symbol of hope and immortality, which are reborn each year when spring arrives and new shoots appear.

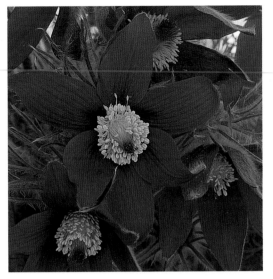

RIGHT The color of the pasqueflower, *Pulsatilla vulgaris*, inspires creativity. Violet is used by therapists to restore energy and strengthen the body's cell structure.

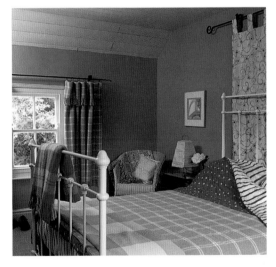

RIGHT Blue creates a feeling of space, and is a good color for a bedroom. It calms tension and brings tranquility, aiding a restful night's sleep.

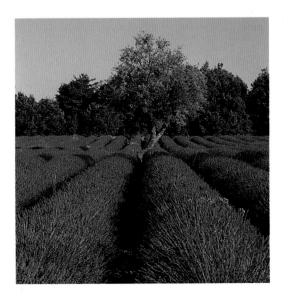

RIGHT A fragrant field of lavender combines blue and violet tones. Blue is inspirational, and mixed with violet it helps to heighten spiritual awareness.

Blue is the color of communication. It is a calming, cooling, relaxing color and so is particularly good for those with flighty energy or a tendency toward overexcitement. Blue is linked to the throat chakra and color healers acknowledge that true communication can only take place in a calm and relaxed atmosphere. Blue is used to treat insomnia, to calm fevers, and to help calm inflammation, irritation, itching, and burns.

Indigo, with its calming and pacifying energy, stimulates the creative and intuitive right brain. Its sedative action means that it is ideal for quelling mental anguish and for harmonizing any physical, mental or spiritual disturbance. This makes it useful in the treatment of insomnia and all nervous disorders. Indigo stimulates the parathyroid and depresses the thyroid and is useful with all types of swellings and bleeding (i.e. nose-bleeds and internal or external hemorrhage). It also stimulates the third eye, improving the powers of insight and intuition.

Violet/purple is the color linked to the crown chakra. It is the color of creativity, inspiration, transformation, enlightenment, and spirituality. It is a powerful calmer of both mind and body and helps one to attune to one's higher spiritual purpose. It is also linked with a sense of self-respect. Violet is often used to treat psychological disorders.

Once you begin to understand and work with color, you will be amazed at the positive effects that changing the colors you wear and have around you can initiate. The power of color is one of the most accessible of all healing energies and one that everyone should learn and understand. Explore this fascinating realm and you will find that the power of color can change your life for the better.

Sound healing

Sound and music form part of the foundation of all social groups throughout the world. Music has the power to evoke deep emotional responses within us and so it follows that the use of sound in healing can be an exceptionally powerful tool. The ancient civilizations understood the power of healing sounds. Three-thousand-year-old Egyptian papyri detail many incantations to cure a wide variety of illnesses. The power of the spoken or sung word has formed one of the basic principles in all religions and spiritual paths.

Sound healing today covers a vast array of therapies and techniques. There is shamanic drumming, trance dance, overtoning, singing bowls, chanting, mantras, meditative music, and ethnic/world music to name but a few. All have some therapeutic effect. Now sound healing is developing in the West as a major, specific therapy with sound healers and teachers

working throughout North America and Europe, running workshops, teaching courses, and allowing anyone to experience the healing power of sound.

The nature of sound

The vibration of any musical note or sound is measured in a scale called hertz (Hz). If the note of middle C is played on a piano, the vibration of that note is 256Hz. This means that the string of the piano is vibrating back and forth 256 times every second. Whenever a note is played, your ear not only hears the vibration of that note, but it also hears notes vibrating above that fundamental note. These other vibrations are called "harmonics" or "overtones." Overtones are responsible for the quality of sound we hear and it is these overtones that allow us to distinguish between the same notes played on different instruments. All

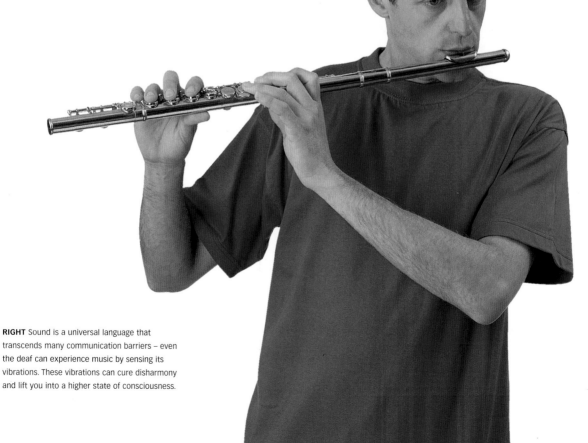

RIGHT Sound is a universal language that transcends many communication barriers – even the deaf can experience music by sensing its vibrations. These vibrations can cure disharmony and lift you into a higher state of consciousness.

instruments produce overtones but different tones are highlighted in different instruments. There are also overtones present in the human voice too; it is these overtones that give our voices their unique characteristics.

An interval is the space between two notes. The most well-known description of the notes of the Western musical scale is "do, re, mi, fa, soh, la, ti, do" a system developed in the eleventh century by the Italian monk Guido D'Arezzo. The interval between the first do and the second do is called an octave. The space between the notes do and re is called "a second" interval, between do and mi is called a third and so on. The words major, minor, augmented and perfect refer to fine tunings where perfect is the normal interval and the others are higher or lower tunings whose interval size is smaller than a second.

Sacred sounding

Sacred sounding, or toning, as it is sometimes called is a very powerful spiritual practice. An individual or a group can practice it and it requires no special vocal skills or training. To experience basic toning all you need is to be able to sing a note. As you sing that note, change the shape of your mouth and listen to how this changes the quality of the note. Try singing the same note while slowly changing the shape to sound the vowels a-e-i-o-u. As you sing, you will naturally begin to notice overtones and harmonics. Allow the resonance of your voice to give power to these vibrations until you feel your whole body vibrating with the note you are singing. Sacred sounding can open, cleanse, and energize the body, mind, and spirit. It can be used to cleanse crystals and to change the energy of places. As you sing, allow the energy of the universe to flow through your voice. Don't be frightened to experiment with different sounds and notes. You will be amazed at the energy you can create.

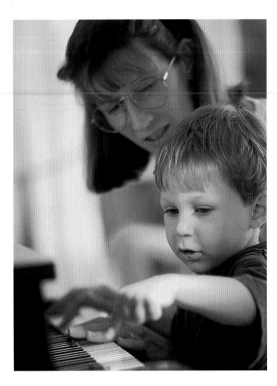

LEFT A child's response to music is spontaneous and energetic. Music therapy is often used to reach children with communication problems or learning difficulties.

THE VIBRATIONAL FREQUENCIES OF HARMONICS

The first 16 harmonics created using middle C as the fundamental note are as follows:

	Note	Interval	Frequency of vibration
1	C	Unison	256Hz
2	C	Octave	512Hz
3	G	Perfect fifth	768Hz
4	C	Octave	1024Hz
5	E	Major third	1280Hz
6	G	Perfect fifth	1536Hz
7	B flat	Minor seventh	792Hz
8	C	Octave	2048Hz
9	D	Major second	2304Hz
10	E	Major third	2560Hz
11	F sharp	Augmented fourth	816Hz
12	G	Perfect fifth	3072Hz
13	A	Minor sixth	3328Hz
14	B flat	Minor seventh	3584Hz
15	B	Major seventh	3840Hz
16	C	Octave	4096Hz

As you can see, a simple note such a middle C creates many vibrations and harmonic overtones of other notes.

Mantras

A mantra is a word or phrase that is repeatedly sung or spoken to induce a spiritually open state of mind. This ancient practice has been used to aid meditation and to evoke the body's own healing energies. Perhaps the most famous of all mantras is the Om. It is a Sanskrit sacred symbol that has been called "the first mantra". It is sounded as an extended "aum" and when repeated can generate some amazing overtones and harmonic resonances that pervade a whole room. Try singing or speaking a mantra for 10 minutes in a silent room either on your own or with friends. The only way to truly understand their power is to experience them firsthand.

The following is a guide to some of the best-known mantras and with a descriptions of how they sound:

The main Hindu mantra: Om (A-U-M, pronounced Ah Hum), the trinity of earth, atmosphere, and heaven.

Hindu healing mantras: Hrim (Hreeemmm) – energizes the throat, Hrum (Hrooommm) – energizes the liver, Hraim (Hraheemmm) – energizes the kidneys, Hraum (Hrowmmm) – energizes the bladder and bowels, and Hra (Hrah) – energizes the heart.

Christian mantra: Alleluia.

Celtic mantra: Awn (Ah...ooh...nn)

Jewish mantra: Shalom – peace.

Islamic mantra: An Nur – God, the light.

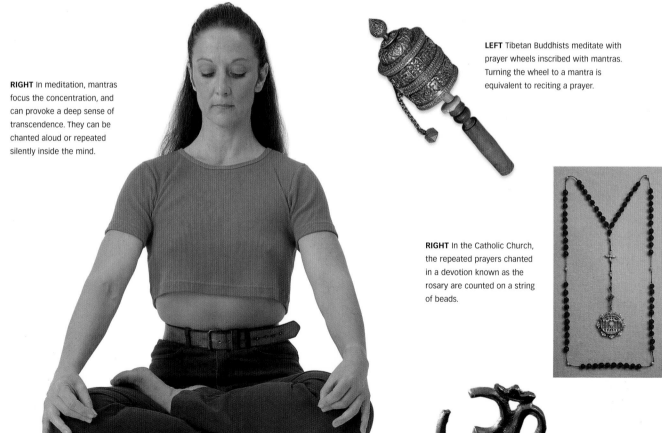

RIGHT In meditation, mantras focus the concentration, and can provoke a deep sense of transcendence. They can be chanted aloud or repeated silently inside the mind.

LEFT Tibetan Buddhists meditate with prayer wheels inscribed with mantras. Turning the wheel to a mantra is equivalent to reciting a prayer.

RIGHT In the Catholic Church, the repeated prayers chanted in a devotion known as the rosary are counted on a string of beads.

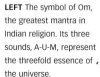

LEFT The symbol of Om, the greatest mantra in Indian religion. Its three sounds, A-U-M, represent the threefold essence of the universe.

THE CHAKRAS AND MUSICAL NOTES

Each of the seven major chakras has a specific note:

To energize each chakra, try singing the specific note into each chakra.
Allow the overtones to resonate until you feel the individual chakra energized.

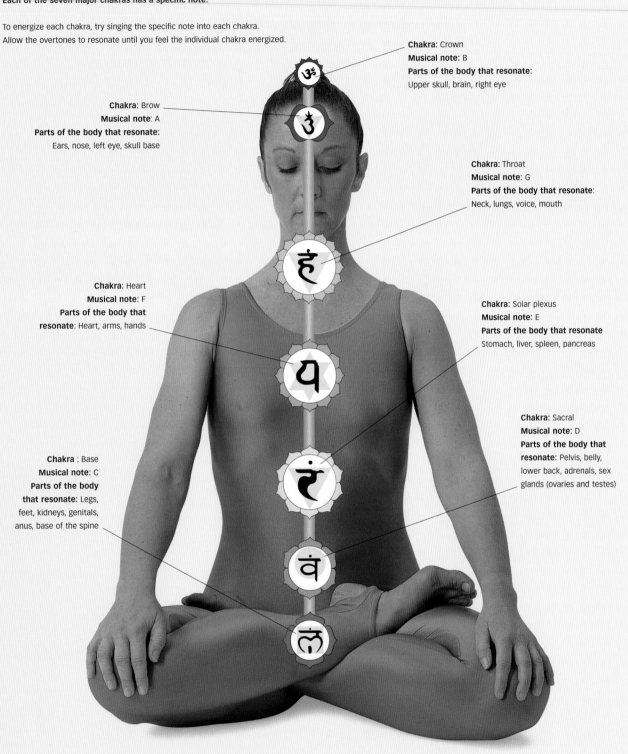

Chakra: Crown
Musical note: B
Parts of the body that resonate:
Upper skull, brain, right eye

Chakra: Brow
Musical note: A
Parts of the body that resonate:
Ears, nose, left eye, skull base

Chakra: Throat
Musical note: G
Parts of the body that resonate:
Neck, lungs, voice, mouth

Chakra: Heart
Musical note: F
**Parts of the body that
resonate:** Heart, arms, hands

Chakra: Solar plexus
Musical note: E
Parts of the body that resonate
Stomach, liver, spleen, pancreas

Chakra: Sacral
Musical note: D
**Parts of the body that
resonate:** Pelvis, belly,
lower back, adrenals, sex
glands (ovaries and testes)

Chakra : Base
Musical note: C
**Parts of the body
that resonate:** Legs,
feet, kidneys, genitals,
anus, base of the spine

Light therapy

It has long been known that sunlight plays a vital role in our moods. In the spring and summer, the whole of creation is alive and vibrant with energy. In the winter much of nature's activity either halts or slows down dramatically.

Humans too are strongly affected by sunlight. It is now known that at least 20 per cent of the light that enters our eyes is not used for seeing, but acts as triggers to the body's endocrine system instructing it on what hormones to produce in what quantity depending on the length and intensity of the sunlight. Shorter daylight hours trigger the production of a hormone called melatonin. Melatonin is known as the sleep hormone because it makes our bodies more sluggish and in need of more sleep. Melatonin's relationship with light and its energy-draining power has also given it the name "Dracula's hormone." It is also the hormone at the root of seasonal affective disorder (SAD).

Melatonin has an enemy, a hormone called serotonin. We naturally produce this energizing hormone in spring and summer and it is this that makes us feel good when the warmer days come. Serotonin is also responsible for strengthening the immune system and improving muscle growth and tone. This fine balance of hormones within the body and their relationship to light has sparked a renewed interest in various forms of light therapy. Perhaps the most remarkable is a therapy called "colored strobe therapy." It uses different colored flashing lights shone into the patient's eyes to treat a variety of illnesses, including anxiety, phobias, depression, learning disorders, hyperactivity, epilepsy, as well as speeding recovery from a stroke. The results have been staggering.

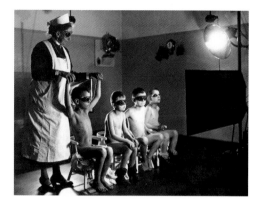

ABOVE Bright white light has been used to maintain health for more than a century. It stimulates the production of vitamin D, the "sunshine vitamin," which strengthens the bones.

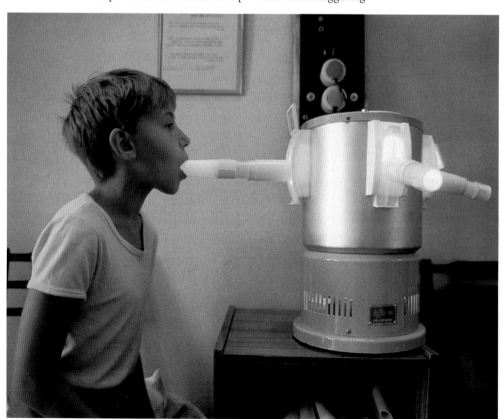

RIGHT Here ultraviolet light is used to treat a child's throat infection. UV rays have an antibacterial effect, and help to heal the skin.

In Britain, Dr David Norton conducted a study treating 17 women with long-standing premenstrual syndrome (PMS) using a red flickering light mask worn by each of the women for 15 minutes each day over four menstrual cycles. Each of the women had been suffering from PMS for more than 10 years. At the end of the study, 12 of the women reported that they were no longer suffering from PMS, one woman abandoned the programme due to increased depression, one showed no change, and the other three showed improvement, but not total eradication of symptoms.

More and more scientists and doctors are beginning to research and use light as a therapeutic aid to health and healing. It is now established that fluorescent lighting is bad for your health. New bulbs that emit full-spectrum light have been shown to improve concentration and reduce stress levels. Research is now being carried out to investigate polarized

light. This is white light that has been split into its individual colors using a prism to form a rainbow. Dr Márta Fenyö runs a clinic in Budapest using polarized light to treat leg ulcers, acne, psoriasis, and sports injuries. She has successfully treated thousands of patients using a drug-free technique called "bio-stimulation," which involves polarized light. Doctors and scientists in Britain are now beginning to study her research.

Light and light-related therapies will undoubtedly grow in strength and popularity as people seek real solutions to their chronic health problems and, who knows, perhaps one day doctors will prescribe 15 minutes of sunbathing instead of reaching for their prescription pads.

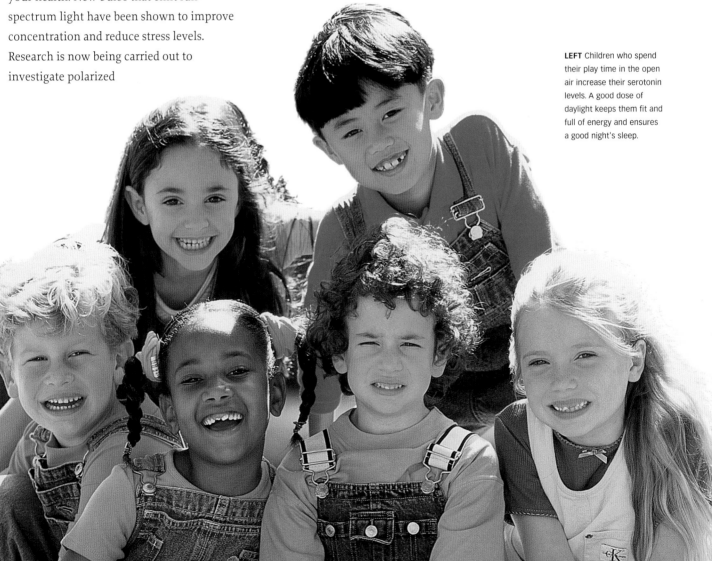

LEFT Children who spend their play time in the open air increase their serotonin levels. A good dose of daylight keeps them fit and full of energy and ensures a good night's sleep.

Final word

It would take at least 20 volumes the size of this book to even begin to properly explain this vast field of energy and energy healing. Clearly, the fact that energy is understood by all ancient cultures and that energy healing is being practiced the entire world over means that it cannot be ignored. It may not provide the answers to all your problems, but it will certainly give you a new perspective and understanding of yourself and the universe around you. The fact that energy is constant and apparently limitless in the universe indicates that the study of energy and energy healing is also without limit.

This book has been designed to give you a taste of this fascinating subject. There is no such thing as an incurable disease and just because Western medicine does not have drugs or surgery that can cure all illnesses does not mean that other therapies will not provide the answer. In the West we have tended to be led to believe that if Western medicine cannot provide answers, the answers do not exist.

It is the birthright of every human being to be happy, healthy, and fulfilled. If you have any kind of illness, do not accept that you just have to live with it. The cure to every disease lies within the person suffering that disease. Energy healing has many powerful therapies and one of them may just provide the answer you are looking for. Search within yourself and in the world at large and you will ultimately find the solution to all your problems. This will only become reality for you if you accept total responsibility for curing yourself. This does not mean that you do not look for outside help. What it does mean is that you remain in charge of your

own healing process and that you never give up searching until you have found happiness, health, and fulfillment.

The field of energy healing is diverse, but if approached with an open mind, it can teach you more about yourself and your health than you can possibly imagine. At the back of this book is a list of contact addresses and the names of therapists that are personally known to the author and recommended by him. This does not mean that they will definitely provide the answers you are seeking, neither does it mean that they are the only people who can help you. The therapists listed are of a high quality and they all work from a perspective of love and respect for all life. If you are interested in any particular field, the resources section will at least provide you with a starting point.

Remember, every experience can be positive and teach you new things if you approach life with a desire to learn and become wiser. Failure is not in falling down, it is in not getting up again. Walk with beauty and the universe will reward you with beauty in return.

Index

Further information

Shen Tao
For a list of shen tao practitioners contact The Shen Tao Foundation, Middle Piccadilly Natural Healing Centre, Holwell, Sherborne, Dorset, DT9 5LW, U.K.

Shamanic essences
For information about shamanic essences contact Sally Hamilton, PO Box 2453, Frome, Somerset, BA11 3YN, U.K. or telephone 01373 812864 during office hours.

Gem and crystal elixirs
High quality elixirs are made by Pegasus Products, PO Box 228, Boulder, Colorado 80306 U.S.A. Tel (303) 667-3019, Andreas Korte, Alpenstrasse 25, D-78262 Gailingen, Germany, GVM, Crystal Herbs, Waverly Lodge, Hoxne, Suffolk, IP21 4AS, U.K. Telephone 01379 642374 or Green Man Trees (address below). The International Flower Essence Repertoire, The Living Tree, Milland, Nr. Liphook, Hampshire, GU30 7JS, U.K. can supply certain gem and crystal elixirs, provide a list of qualified Vibrational Medicine Practitioners, and advise on the latest developments in the field. For courses in Vibrational Medicine contact IFVM, Middle Piccadilly Natural Healing Centre, Holwell, Sherbourne, Dorset, DT9 5LW or Mandragora, c/o Green Man Trees, 2 Kerswell Cottages, Exminster, Devon, EX6 8AY, U.K.

Ayurveda
A list of qualified Ayurvedic practitioners can be found by consulting the Association of Ayurvedic Practitioners, 7 Ravenscourt Avenue, London, NW11 0SA, U.K.

Homeopathy
For more information about homeopathy contact Society of Homeopaths, 2 Artizan Road, Northampton, NN1 4HU, U.K. Phone 01604 621400. Email:societyofhomeopaths@btinternet.com. For medical homeopaths contact British Homeopathic Association, 27a Devonshire Street, London W1N 1RJ, U.K. Telephone 0171 935 2163.

Radionics
To find out more about radionics or for a list of qualified practitioners contact The Radionic Association. Baerlein House, Goose Green, Deddington, Banbury, Oxon. OX15 0SZ, U.K.

RESOURCES LIST

Practitioners
The following U.K. practitioners have all contributed information for this book.

Andy Baggott Dip.Ac. Dip.CST.
Little Acre Natural Healing Centre, PO Box 2453, Frome, Somerset, BA11 3YN, U.K. Email: andy@celtlodg.globalnet.co.uk

Traditional Chinese Medicine and Macrobiotic Nutrition, Traditional Herbalism, Craniosacral Therapy and Celtic Shamanism.

Les Martin and Marloes Van Eck
Tel/Fax: 01761 435107
Macrobiotic Dietary Therapists.

Catriona Cusick Riley Tel: 01296 393013.
Email: CCUSICK4@aol.com
Acupuncture, Craniosacral Therapy, Herbal Medicine, Bach Flower Remedies, Kinesiology, Macrobiotic Dietary Therapy, Chi Kung exercise.

Ina Jansen ISPA, BAPTAC, ITEC. Tel/Fax: 0181 940 5341
Aromatherapy (Micheline Arcier trained) and Natural Beauty Therapy.

Clare G. Harvey Middle Piccadilly, Holwell, Nr. Sherbourne, Dorset, DT9 5EL, U.K. Tel: 01963 323038. Also at The Hale Clinic, 7 Park Crescent, London. Tel: 0171 631 0604. Vibrational Medicine and Flower Remedies.

Eliana Harvey Middle Piccadilly, Holwell, Nr. Sherbourne, Dorset, DT9 5EL, U.K. Tel: 01963 323038. Shen Tao and Shamanka (wise woman) training.

Sheila Gore DSH 8 Cheap Street, Frome, Somerset, BA11 1BN, U.K. Tel: 01373 473334. Licenced Homeopath.

Sally Hamilton Almadel Healing Centre, c/o PO Box 2453, Frome, Somerset, BA11 1YN, U.K. Vibrational Medicine and Animal Healing.

ORGANIZATIONS

Alternative Medicine Information
Jackie Wooton, M.Ed.
Fax: (001) 301 340-1936.
Email: jackiew@clark.net
Web Site:
http://www.clark.net/pub/AltMedInfo/ USA

American Association for Oriental Medicine
4101 Lake Boone Trail
Suite 201
Raleigh NC 27607, USA
Tel: (919) 787-5181
Web site:
http://www.aaom.org/aahome.htm

National Acupuncture and Oriental Medicine Alliance
14637 Starr Road SE
Olalla WA 98359, USA
Tel: (206) 851-6896
Email:76143.2061@compuserve.com

Ayurvedic Institute
11311 Menaul NE
Suite A
Alburquerque NM 87112, USA
Tel: (505) 291-9698
Fax: (505) 294-7572

George Ohsawa Macrobiotic Foundation
1511 Robinson Street
Oroville
California 95965, USA
Tel: (916) 533-7702

The Kushi Institute (for Macrobiotics)
PO Box 7
Becket MA 01233, USA

National Holistic Institute
5900 Hollis St
Suite J
Emeryville CA 94608-2008, USA
Register of Chinese Herbal Medicine
21 Warbreck Road
London W10 8NS, U.K.

Association of Systematic Kinesiology
39 Browns Road
Surbiton
Surrey KT5 8ST, U.K.

U.K. Polarity Therapy Association
Monomark House
27 Old Gloucester Street
London WC1N 3XX, U.K.

Craniosacral Therapy Association of Great Britain
8 Warren Road
Colliers Wood
London SW19 2HX, U.K.

Institute for Complementary Medicine
PO Box 194
London SE16 1QZ, U.K.

The National Federation of Spiritual Healers (NFSH)
Old Manor Farm Studio
Church Street
Sunbury-on-Thames
Middlesex TW16 6RG, U.K.

Alternative Health Information Bureau
12 Upper Station Road
Radlett
Hertfordshire WD7 3BX, U.K.

International Association of Reiki
Mari Hall
Lesni 14
46001 Liberec
Czech Republic
Email: reiki@Lbc.pvtnet.cz